THE
BETTER BACK
BOOK

Simple Exercises
for the
Prevention and Care
of Back Pain

CONSTANCE A. BEAN

WILLIAM MORROW AND COMPANY, INC.   NEW YORK

Library of Congress Cataloging-in-Publication Data

Bean, Constance. A.
    The better back book / by Constance A. Bean.
        p.   cm.
    ISBN 0-688-07915-6
    1. Backache—Exercise therapy. I. Title.
RQ771.B217B43   1989
617'.56—dc19   88-12925
                                                        CIP

Printed in the United States of America

First Edition

1 2 3 4 5 6 7 8 9 10

BOOK DESIGN AND LINE ART BY JAYE ZIMET

ACKNOWLEDGMENTS

I wish to thank Lisa Drew, Senior Editor at William Morrow and Company, for the special care she took and especially to express my appreciation for her vision.

I want to thank Eva Statz, M.D., for reading this manuscript and for her interest in this book.

The models for the book who were so generous with their time were Carolyn Wagoner, Michael Sylvester, and David Bean.

The photographers who provided expert attention to detail were Robert Ruscansky of Needham, Massachusetts, for the two male models, and Dudley of Honolulu, Hawaii, for the female model.

Also invaluable was the feedback from participants in the Take Care of Your Back Program at M.I.T. during the past four years.

Constance A. Bean

CONTENTS

Acknowledgments   5

One. Back Problems and Puzzlements: The Issues and the Questions   9

Two. Back Attack: Now What?   17

Three. Causes of Back Pain   32

Four. Getting Moving   52

Five. What Next? Level One Back Exercises   63

Six. On Your Way: Level Two Back Exercises   78

Seven. Up-and-About Back Protection   92

Eight. Level Three: The Icing on the Cake   105

Nine. Would a Health Club Help?   143

Ten. Pregnancy and Afterward   155

Eleven. Medicine and Your Back   166

Twelve. Keeping What You've Got   200

Appendixes
Glossary   211
Back Organizations   215
Bibliography   217

Index   225

CHAPTER ONE

BACK PROBLEMS AND PUZZLEMENTS: THE ISSUES AND THE QUESTIONS

☐

Back pain is largely a preventable problem. Yet the chances of having severe backache or back trouble at some time during your life are high, as high as 85 percent. All sources agree that the figure is at least 80 percent. According to the American Institute for Preventive Medicine, about eighty million people in the United States are currently coping with back pain, yet 80 percent, or four out of five of these backaches, could have been avoided.

Backache is the most common work injury today, usually striking people between the ages of twenty and fifty. Statistics show that about 60 percent of those with severe, incapacitating pain, whether it is known to be work-related or not, will have another attack within two years.

Backache is the major cause of disability in people under forty-five and is second only to the common cold in terms of time lost from work. In addition, there are many more, for whom there are no statistics, who experience occasional tightness or soreness in their backs. They feel their tiredness in their backs. And those who have had no complaints of backache? If they ignore basic back care as a vital part of their ongoing health concerns, they set themselves up, unknowingly in most cases, for a future back attack.

A sedentary life-style is a major risk factor. The underlying cause of 80 percent of back pain is alleged to be lack of exercise. This statement should be changed to read "lack of appropriate exercise." Golf, tennis, or softball in themselves offer little protection. Sports such as these may even be the precipitating cause of back pain. Gymnastics and crew activities carry substantial risk for back injury and pain.

Back distress may happen once, or many times. It may be a recurrent theme throughout life. Sometimes you can connect it with an accident or injury. You know you fell on the ski slope or a car slammed into yours, and afterward, perhaps immediately or maybe a while later, you became aware of stiffness and pain. You knew that you were in difficulty, that you needed help. You were in pain and it would not go away.

More likely the pain seemed to come from nowhere. There is nothing you could remember to account for the fact that you found yourself partially or even completely disabled, and for an indeterminate time as well. You may have said, "I sneezed and my back went out." Or, "I started to turn around and suddenly I got this pain in my back." Maybe you had some discomfort off and on, but it got worse, not better, and you struggled to recall whether you lifted something that might have been too heavy. You may have felt somewhat guilty as well, even though you had no way of knowing how much weight your back is prepared to accept.

Finding yourself in pain for no apparent reason can be disconcerting, if not frightening. You become aware that your life might be largely and to an uncertain extent out of your control for a while or even forever. Taking off even a couple of days usually requires real planning. Everything is affected—studies, job, child care, social life, shopping, and all the myriad things that just have to be done.

When you acknowledge that you are definitely in trouble, you call for medical attention. You call someone— your internist, an orthopedist, or your health maintenance organization. You find someone to drive you to a walk-in clinic or hospital emergency room. Your friend suggests a chiropractor. Perhaps you go to a sports medicine clinic.

Typically the result of your visit is that you learn that "We really don't know what causes back pain." You are reminded that humans originally walked on all fours and that the upright position for walking has contributed to back problems ever since.

You may be advised to spend two weeks on bed rest, with shower and bathroom visits only, and perhaps not even those. Because current studies show lack of increased benefit with prolonged bed rest, this makes it more, not less, difficult to know what recommendations to anticipate. You may be told to stay in bed until there has been no pain for twenty-four or forty-eight hours while you remain at rest, whatever length of time that may be. Applications of heat may be suggested. In a couple of days you may be fine.

You will most likely be given a list of three or four standard back exercises to do. Also included may be a sheet on "body mechanics" to assist you in the future to lift properly, to sit, to drive, and to stand so you might prevent future injury. Perhaps you will be given a prescription for a pain reliever to be filled if you need it. Your emotions and the practical difficulties you face are not addressed. You are sent on your way.

Oftentimes you leave the office feeling you do not know much more than when you came in, and you have further questions as well. You are unclear as to when in the recovery process to start exercising, how often to do the exercises, and you are not even exactly sure that you understand how to do them correctly. It seems bizarre to have in hand an exercise prescription when you can barely get out of your chair.

You wonder if walking on two feet instead of on all fours may have doomed you to a life of worrying about your back. You think you will never again be able to move furniture or carry your own suitcases. Will you ever be able to trust your back again?

You may have other feelings as well. Your doctor's possible apparent indifference to your plight may be anything but reassuring. You know that there may be a couple of days, a couple of weeks, or even months in bed. There are no guarantees about recovery. Your view of your future appears murky at best. Yet it seems that your legitimate concerns elicit scant response from the world of medicine. You wonder if there are more answers than you have been given. Around you a cloud seems to drift, a conspiracy of silence. The message seems to be "never mind the whys and the wherefores."

Another scenario is possible if the pain is acute or has been a problem in the past. Your health care provider may suggest X rays. You may feel relieved, or you may hesitate. If you are pregnant, X rays will not be done. In any case, a request should be made that a lead shield be used to help protect the reproductive organs and genetic material. More discussion of this point is included in Chapter Eleven, "Medicine and Your Back."

Sometimes a series of back X rays is a prerequisite to being seen. The physician wishes to rule out spinal tumors and view the general configuration of the spine. Soft tissues such as muscles and tendons cannot be seen, but the physician does have a base line by which to evaluate future changes.

The X rays may show abnormality. There may be aberrations in the bony structure of the spine that are considered to be out of the range of normal. There may be narrowing of the "disc spaces," showing compression of the soft, cartilagelike tissue material between the vertebrae. But narrowed disc spaces are considered to be a normal accompaniment to aging, as are certain bone changes. Complicating this scenario is the fact that sometimes certain abnormalities will present themselves on an X-ray film, but the patient has no back pain. Or the patient has pain, but there is nothing particularly unusual about the X-ray films. Often there is no direct correlation between the back X-ray findings and the patient's symptoms. The most common problems, often not even an acute disc injury, do not show up on the X ray.

Seldom will X-ray results change the course of treatment. However, certain symptoms such as bladder problems or severe pain and numbness in the leg may elicit discussion of the need for surgery (see Chapter Eleven).

In most cases you are informed that there is no known cause of your pain. And you cannot document your pain. You remember stories of alleged fraudulent insurance claims and wonder if your story that you cannot get into your car and drive will sound credible. If you do make the attempt to remain mobile, you do not even know whether you could harm yourself or delay your recovery. Your friends may tell you that back pain can even be psychological in origin, resulting from stress in your life. Your medical provider may suggest this also, if a series of visits appears to produce no improvement.

What you have learned so far is hardly guaranteed to reduce your feelings of vulnerability and helplessness. Your healthy body has betrayed you. You feel out of control, and, to a large extent, you are.

On the other hand, you receive the message, even though probably not stated directly, that your recovery depends on you. No one else can do it, whatever "it" is. When you learn what "it" is, you may find that the steps you take and the ensuing results may enhance dramatically your self-esteem and self-confidence. There are individual differences and needs, but with some guiding principles you can be active in planning your own recovery from the moment you take to your bed, and, yes, you can act to prevent back problems in the future.

Admittedly all of the answers on back pain and back problems are not yet in. The available literature can help, yet have contradictions and leave questions. Medical answers are frequently unsatisfactory or necessarily incomplete, leaving patients insecure about the recovery program on which they are embarking. Because much of the needed research has not yet been done, many of the recommendations come from the reported experiences of patients.

Health care providers, on the other hand, find counseling back patients to be difficult, not only because of the shortage of time allotted for clinical appointments but also because they have almost as many uncertainties as do the patients, and each patient situation is somewhat different from others. Assessment is difficult, as is analyzing the patient's life-style. Many doctors find the treatment of back pain patients to be unrewarding at best. Answering a patient's questions is time-consuming and fraught with uncertainty, often leaving the patient unclear whether to rest or to exercise or to try to go to work or to embark on a swimming program!

The health care provider's comments must necessarily be general and will be colored by the background and training provided by the particular specialty of the provider, whether athletic trainer, internal medicine specialist, physical therapist, or other. As with such topics as sexuality, nutrition, and exercise, back care falls under more than one umbrella. The frequent wait-and-see response from providers may be wise, but it is often frustrating to patients.

Acute back pain usually does tend to get better within a few days or weeks. Nobody can tell, or even guess how long. This is not your standard disease entity with a predictable sequence of events. There is wide variability in back pain episodes and in the courses they take. It is often said that back patients usually get better no matter what is done, the implication being that patients should feel free to try whatever works for them.

Most back exercise programs, whether exercise classes or handout sheets, cannot undertake to give you a strong, flexible body or even a strong back, which is what you need to be pain-free. Helpful suggestions are offered but generally are inadequate for those seeking detailed information. Some suggestions are controversial. Providers state repeatedly that exercise programs seldom are followed after back pain subsides, thereby lowering their incentives to develop comprehensive back fitness programs, which require gathering interdisciplinary resources from physical therapy, neurology, physiology, sports medicine, orthopedics, and others. The lack of patient compliance relates, too, to the high level of back pain recurrence.

This book aims to give you a practical, straightforward, easy-to-follow program that you will want to adopt, more as a stress-relieving break than an unwelcome chore or burden. Important exercises have been included, and unnecessary or potentially harmful exercises explained.

Taking care of your back involves more than the traditional rest, more than practicing sit-ups, and more than applications of heat. With the exception of heat these may constitute your first steps, but there is a longer view. Progress is measured by observing that your pain-free time increases, you can stand longer, walk farther, sit longer, lift more, and move your body safely in ways you have not previously dared.

If your back does not respond to your care, you will want to know what happens next. There are numerous controversies in this area, too, and a variety of options. Your aim is to be an informed participant in the decision-making process. For most people, with certain exceptions, the conservative posture is adopted. Rest and exercise, not tests and surgery, comprise the treatment. The challenge of finding the answers is yours.

Because the approach in most cases needs to be one of health promotion rather than one of medical treatment, you will necessarily be making most of the decisions about life-style changes. This can be truly awe-inspiring when you fear that one false move may make things worse, and even more so if you have not previously been an active participant in your health care. Achieving success in eliminating back pain and overcoming your subsequent feelings of vulnerability can increase your confidence in your ability to take care of yourself. As with so many other health issues, such as cardiovascular problems and lung disease, self-care is of prime importance, and in the end it can be an empowering life experience.

CHAPTER TWO

BACK ATTACK:
NOW WHAT?

☐

Before looking at charts il-
lustrating the structure of your back and discovering just
how vulnerable to injury your back is, focus your attention
on your back and exactly how it feels. (If your back is
currently hurting, you need to be able to describe it clearly
to your doctor.) Often descriptions of back pain are sur-
prisingly vague. If you can articulate your problem, this
will help you to plan your treatment and assist, perhaps
indirectly, in evaluating your improvement as you progress through your back fitness and body strengthening
program. What is the problem as you see it?

Instead of attempting to deny the pain, fearing it, or
reaching for the aspirin, try to look at it as a signal that you
need to do something for your back. Try, if possible, to
understand the pain as much as possible, to see it as
valuable feedback in helping you assess what your back
needs from you. What helps your back? What seems to
make it worse?

Think quietly and carefully when you first noticed the pain. Is it sharp or dull? Exactly where do you feel it? Do you feel it intermittently or all the time? Do you feel it most when you must remain standing for a period of time? What happens when you sit? Exactly where does the pain seem to be in your back? How extensive is it? Does it extend to your leg? How far down your leg? Is it worse in the morning or as the day wears on? Does your back feel as though it had "seized up" on you, making motion difficult or even impossible? Has this happened in the past? Can you determine possible causes of your back pain? If you have had one or more "back attacks" in the past, are they becoming more frequent? The answers you give to yourself or your health care provider may not change significantly what you do for your back, but they may help you get in better touch with the problem as you gather your resources to initiate the process of resolving your back pain. Keep track of YOUR back story!

The pain may be the result of escalating muscle tension in your back combined with postural problems and weak abdominal muscles. It may be the result of an injury from years back that you no longer remember. Athletic trainers state that orthopedic injuries tend to repeat if the problem is not resolved. A temporary backache felt while sitting on an airplane but that is relieved when you walk off the plane may be a warning that some preventive measures are in order.

On the other hand, you may know that there is no question about it. You may not have a choice whether to attend one more meeting or have one more go at your neighborhood health club. You have to call in sick at work for today, tomorrow, and maybe longer, maybe for weeks, even if you have never, to your knowledge, had a previous back problem.

The first step in conservative treatment is pain relief achieved by resting in the horizontal position. Your physician might send you to the hospital for tests, or to ensure bed rest. Changes in hospital regulations regarding diagnosis and insurance reimbursement make this less likely than formerly.

Typically you will be in your your own bed at home with feelings of isolation, frustration, and uncertainty, alone with your pain, although that may be less of a problem once you become horizontal.

BED REST: YES, HOW TO DO IT!

Achieving bed rest is often difficult and stressful. Almost paradoxically, it is a kind of enforced vacation. Yet it requires active planning. The need for taking control is combined with unaccustomed feelings of dependency because, usually, some assistance is required from one or more people in your life. Your body has let you down. The reality is that you have lost a little or a lot of your independence for an unpredictable period of time. At the same time, by finding this assistance and learning to resolve your back problem, you are "taking charge" perhaps more than ever seemed necessary before.

The foundation for a healthy back is a firm mattress, but the old idea that it must be hard has become obsolete, as has the suggestion that backs are helped by lying on a blanket on the floor. Hard surfaces will tend to cause muscle spasm and pain. A three- or four-inch foam pad on the floor or platform can be used.

In use for years has been the "bed board," a piece of half-inch or three-quarter-inch plywood placed under the mattress if it is soft. If your mattress rests on a platform, as with a platform bed, you need no further support whether your mattress is foam or innerspring, whatever its degree of firmness. The springs are more often the problem than the mattress.

Water beds are fine, but there is no need to seek one out if you don't already have one. Opinions on water beds for back problems are mixed but generally favorable. Pressure on your back is eliminated. Yet the heavier parts of your body sink lower, perhaps changing body alignment. You have to be the judge. Many people like them. But a water bed with wave motion is considered unsuitable, especially if it is shared with another person. You can discuss your individual situation with your medical care provider.

There is more. You will need to move about in bed, and you don't want to have to keep remaking the bed to remain comfortable. The bottom sheet should, of course, be contoured, and many people find a comforter easier to manage than blankets that don't stay tucked in. Keep warm enough to allow your muscles to relax.

Your pillow should be flat enough so that you can lie on your side and allow your body to remain in a horizontal position. You will need another pillow, not too plump, to wedge against your back or between your knees when you lie on your side.

HOW DO I LIE?

Lying flat on your back, called the supine position, has long been disparaged by medical providers and back-sufferers alike because it promotes back muscle spasm, but the back position works well if you modify it by supporting your raised knees on pillows, or if you draw up your knees with your feet resting flat on the bed. This position places your back in correct alignment and begins to give your back muscles the stretch they need and may have lost. For some people this position initially causes pain, even with raised knees, because the muscles are severely contracted in spasm, or because the weight of the body on the back tends to cause soreness and spasm. If the back position with raised knees causes pain, lie instead on your side.

When your knees are raised, your back muscles can relax, whereas if your knees are straight, the back muscles tend to shorten. This is especially true if the abdominal muscles are relaxed or don't have the strength to hold your back in a position that allows those muscles to relax. If you stand with locked knees, just as when you recline with outstretched legs, your back muscles tend to shorten. In the raised-knee back-lying position the pressure on the discs of your back is barely one third of what it is when you stand, less than in any other position you could choose.

When you lie on your side, the forces on your spine are about 75 percent of what they are when you stand. By placing a pillow between your knees you help to keep the strain and pain away from your top hip, and your back remains in better alignment, not twisted. The pillow also reminds you to keep your body horizontal, not raised into a slant. The size of the pillow you need depends on the width of your hips and the thickness of your thighs. If your hips are narrow and your thighs are large, you may not need to use a pillow. Keep your knees flexed (bent).

For those who can sleep only on their stomachs, and no other way, the disappointing news is that this prone position increases the arch of the back. The back muscles then are shortened, and this is conducive to back muscle spasm. If you are currently in pain the chances of your being able to lie on your stomach are remote indeed, just one more piece of evidence that the state of your back has reined in another accustomed pleasure. Later on, even if not in the midst of a fresh new back attack, you can try this position and make it work for you by placing a pillow under your waist and upper abdomen to straighten out your spine. Placing an arm under your abdomen may serve the same purpose. Those with a large abdomen may not need a pillow. Some back books suggest the prone position as a way of strengthening back muscles, but for many it causes pain for a very long time, for many months, and can never be used except for short intervals. There are better ways of strengthening back muscles.

This prone position tends to arch, or hyper-extend, your back. The extended back position causes spinal bones to be bent back on each other to produce stress on joints and muscles. Before you can lie prone, the abdominals must be strong enough to help assure that the back is not excessively arched. The back muscles need first to get out of spasm and then to gain strength.

The fact that you can try it later may offer you a ray of hope. With a strong back, chances are that in the future you can spend, safely and painlessly, stretches of time lying on your stomach.

THE COMFORTS OF HOME

Most bedridden people want a telephone within easy reach. They feel more in control and safer when they can contact the outside world. Hearing a telephone ringing elsewhere in the house is not conducive to reducing anxiety levels when you know you cannot get up to answer it. Being able to receive support from friends and remaining in contact with the outside world in general, whether it be your office, the plumber, your family, or your congressman, allows you to feel that you are indeed still a presence in your world. You can accomplish many of the "to do's" on your list, or not, as you decide.

Although you can try to read in bed, the usual propped, pillows-behind-your-back reading position is neither recommended nor usually comfortable. A variety of ingenious methods for propping books has been tried.

Another aid is a television set near your bed, preferably with a remote control. Even if you do not normally spend your days watching reruns of the classic sitcoms, the talk shows, or the soap operas, as you find the pace of your days remarkably slowed and your calendar almost entirely clear, television may help keep you distracted and relaxed.

Or you can shut off the set and actually have time in your day to think, or listen to music, or look out the window. Because you do not expect to have this happen to you ever again, you might almost savor these days. At least you can try.

How will you eat? If you are alone in your house during the day you will probably welcome lunch, already prepared by someone else, within easy reach of your bed. This can be fruit, cheese, raw vegetables, bread, and sandwiches with fillings that require no refrigeration; also thermoses of milk, tea, or coffee. You cannot really sit up to eat, so you choose food that does not easily spill. Soups have to be drunk from a cup. Lie on your side to eat, raising your head as you need to.

Think twice before you attempt to damp your depression by eating extra amounts of calorie-dense foods supplying little nourishment, such as cookies and pastry. Lying in bed makes it easy to pick up extra pounds. Bed rest uses only about a third of the calories you would burn in an active day. If you carry more than a few pounds of extra weight, especially in the abdominal area, it is considered a significant factor in the incidence of back pain, both the initial episode and recurrence. Ten extra pounds on the abdomen results in one hundred extra pounds of pressure on the cushioning discs between the bony vertebrae of your back. Why? Because it deepens the spine's normal curve as the buttocks push out to compensate for the abdominal weight. It is easy to see why pregnancy requires attention to a back exercise program.

You know what you like to eat. You may be into alfalfa sprouts or big Macs. Friends may bring cheesecake or other goodies to cheer you up. However temporary your bed rest, if you eat an extra five hundred calories each day above what you need, you might well gain a pound at the end of each week. Five hundred calories equal about one dessert.

Care of yourself in other ways depends on your individual situation. You will want toothbrush, toothpaste, water, and dental floss by your bedside; perhaps also a washcloth, brush, and comb. These help to avoid the need to climb out of bed unnecessarily.

Can you get up to take a shower? The hot shower may help to relieve muscle spasms, but standing may be difficult. A soak in the tub may be more in line with your needs. To avoid slipping or tripping, move slowly and carefully.

People have used bedpans, bottles, or jars to collect urine. Some people have even made their trips to the bathroom on all fours. It is hard to know how much the upright position may increase back pain or delay recovery, especially at first. Even with acute, disabling back pain you will probably get up occasionally for a few minutes. This depends on your back situation and the advice of your physician.

"ICE IT"

If you think you may have overstressed your back—if, for example, you twisted as you lifted a shovelful of snow, or slipped and fell—most physicians, nurses, and athletic trainers now suggest ice, not heat, within the first twenty minutes and periodically for the first day or two after the injury. It is felt that cold applications help to prevent bleeding from small muscle tears and prevent the accumulation of fluid and resultant nerve irritation within the tissues. To avoid injury to the skin, do not apply ice directly without a cloth or other covering.

A bag of ice, or even a bag of frozen peas, a frozen steak, or immersing your back in a few inches of cold water in your bathtub for a couple of minutes may help.

It is hard to know. Ice tends to relieve the perception of pain as well as the immediate cause, in this case tissue swelling. Of course, often you don't know for a few hours or even until the next day that you have an injury. If you feel you have done something to risk your back you could use ice as a possible preventive measure. Even though heat may appear infinitely more appealing, when in doubt, "ice it."

"USE HEAT"

Later, after a day or two, heat helps to relax muscles and thereby relieve pain. Lie on your side with your small pillow between your knees. Moist heat, as with a hot water bottle wrapped in a wet towel, or the use of a hydroculator sold in drugstores, is more helpful than the dry heat of a heating pad. Using a hydroculator is more effort than many people like. It looks like a life jacket and requires heating in boiling water. With moist heat you will need extra towels and plastic sheeting to prevent finding yourself lying in a damp bed.

Suggested, usually, is about fifteen minutes of heat one, two, or three times a day. Too much, it is sometimes said, could weaken the muscles of your back. Actually, heat encourages swelling. Muscles can only be weakened by lack of use, lack of nutrition, or a disease condition. Overuse of heat may delay starting an exercise program and therefore result in muscle weakness. Concentrate on relaxing your back muscles against the comforting heat to relieve pain resulting from muscle spasm.

A folded towel under your waist is also suggested to enhance the relaxation of your back muscles as you lie on your side, to maintain the proper alignment of your spine, especially if your hips are much larger than your waist. The purpose is to prevent your waist from sagging in the direction of the bed surface.

ASKING QUESTIONS

You have made yourself as comfortable as possible, but already you are looking ahead. What will be the game plan for your recovery? Many people keep a clipboard and paper, a thick pad of notepaper, or a notebook within reach. A pencil is often easier to use than a pen as you lie flat or nearly so. You have questions to ask of your doctor. Your questions may not all be asked at this time. People have differing needs and problems associated with their common problem of back pain.

You cannot help but have concerns. You don't know whether pregnancy somehow damaged your back forever, or whether the problem is your chair at work, or the staggering amount of stress you are experiencing as you juggle your innumerable and sometimes conflicting responsibilities. Perhaps you may have been so intent on completing a task or important project that you cannot even remember when the pain started, or you pushed through the pain in an effort to finish painting your walls, writing your report, or repairing your car. Back pain may be more disabling than a broken leg. You do not know what caused it, and you cannot demonstrate or prove that you have it. With a broken bone you at least know the nature of the injury and can have reasonable expectations about your return to normal life. Is back pain something you might even have to learn to live with?

What you tell your medical care provider about what you feel and the history you provide will affect the answers you receive and the tests that may be done. As you consider what to do next, the following questions are offered as a checklist.

1. **When may I come in for an appointment? This may depend on appointment availability, but the doctor may also suggest a few days of rest, per-**

haps to avoid the possibility of increasing the pain by taking the trip to his or her office. But still, if the problem is acute, as you describe your symptoms, an immediate visit may be indicated, certainly if an accident has been involved. If the receptionist is making the decision to delay the appointment, you will want to inquire if this person is taking medical responsibility. At this point the receptionist will usually put you straight through to the physician. In most cases no specific treatment is indicated and there may be no urgent need for an immediate appointment.

2. Should I drive myself to the appointment? Driving, sitting, climbing stairs, and standing may all be very uncomfortable or very painful. It is possible to be driven while lying on your side on the backseat. You can wait for the doctor while lying down somewhere, anywhere, including an empty examining room table. Many people are extremely tense in addition to their pain, fearing that they are doing further damage by embarking on this initial trip to the doctor's.

3. Do I need to rest my back? Does this mean bed rest? If so, for how long? How will I know when or how long I can be up?

4. What does this mean, bed rest? How complete should this be? Can I get my own meals? Take showers? Go to the bathroom? Sit up in bed? Are there guidelines I should follow to know when I can increase my activity? Should I apply heat to my back? If so, how often and for how long?

5. Do you have information on the possible cause or causes of my pain and on the possible nature of the injury? Is there any indication that this might be associated with a disc problem or structural problem in my back such as scoliosis or something else? You want serious answers, not flip opinions

about your advancing age or too much tennis, and not an impatient put-down such as "That's an impossible question." True, the physician may not know the answer, but expect to receive whatever information is available and that a careful history will be taken.

6. When should I check back with you? Should I call or come in to see you? Are there circumstances that would indicate that I should call you sooner?

7. What about exercise programs, and when will I start to do back exercises? What pamphlets do you have that describe exercises, and will you plan to show me how these are done? Do you also have instruction sheets on ways of avoiding future back injury?

These seven question groups are the basic ones. You may have others you wish to add to your list. If at a later time medical interventions such as tests or the unlikely event of possible surgery are indicated, you will have further questions; an additional series of inquiries are included later in this book. Do not expect definitive answers to all of these seven question groups, but listen to the answers and try to assess whether they appear relevant to your situation and whether you feel that the communication between you and your doctor is sufficient to ensure a working partnership in the resolution of your problem.

If you think your back pain may be related to a work-related injury, you must seek medical care as soon as possible. Check right away with your personnel or safety office, especially if it becomes clear that you will lose time from your job. You need medical documentation and paperwork done.

If you have been in an accident not related to your job, prompt medical attention is also necessary. Records must be kept for insurance purposes. In either instance make it clear to the receptionist that you need to be seen right away. Often back pain is not seen as urgent but as the chronic and frustrating problem it usually is.

As you plan your route to recovery, ask yourself a series of questions. If you feel discouraged at some of your answers, this does not mean that the "wrong answers" are related to your back pain. They do help you, and perhaps your doctor, too, assess where you are now. Your back pain challenges you to upgrade your health promotion efforts. And unlike, for example, your cholesterol-lowering program, your salt reduction attempts, or your quit-smoking program, you see results yourself in terms of less or no pain.

SELF-ASSESSMENT
QUESTIONNAIRE

1. Am I significantly overweight? Do I have a protruding abdomen?

2. Do I sit a substantial number of hours each day without periodic breaks for walking, stretching, and position changes?

3. Does my chair have support for my lower back, and is the chair low enough for my feet to rest comfortably on the floor? Does the chair rock back to ease and vary pressures on the spine? When I lean forward, do I remember to place my elbows on the desk while keeping my back straight, neither hollowed nor curved?

4. Do I regularly stand for long periods, especially in tight shoes, or in the case of women, in shoes with raised heels? Do I often wear sandals that slip and slide on my feet, resulting in tensing of back muscles?

5. Does my job or hobby require that I perform repetitive motions using the same muscle groups?

6. Do I lift objects and loads at sporadic intervals without knowing just how to lift and without taking the time to recognize how my back feels?

7. Is my mattress comfortable? What about the chair in which I often doze for long stretches of time in front of the television set?

8. Is the seat of my car positioned correctly? Is there adequate support for my lower back in the seat of my car?

9. How do I habitually stand? Is the hollow of my lower back exaggerated, or is it tipped so far in the opposite direction that my lower back tends to curve outward?

10. How do I assess my level of fitness? Am I engaged in an exercise program, and if so, what kind? Do I adhere to it regularly or sporadically? Do I include more than one type of physical activity? Do I get expert information when I engage in a new sport or fitness program?

11. Do I feel that I can take time out to relax? Do I often or occasionally practice the "relaxation response" in which I consciously relax each of my voluntary muscles? Do I take "time out" during the day for myself? How do I assess my stress level? Is the level of stress I feel a comfortable one, providing challenges I enjoy? Or do I feel uncomfortable and burdened?

12. Do I recall previous episodes of back pain, and if so, what, if anything, did I do about it? What was helpful? Do I recall any specific injury in the recent or distant past that might have contributed to my present back pain? Remember that it is often

difficult to relate cause and effect, and in any case, your recollections may not affect significantly what you do now.

13. If I feel that I would like another opinion, what other medical resources might I tap to assess my condition and add to my information about myself?

The above self-assessment gives you an initial indication of risk factors that may be involved in your back pain, or back pain you might have in the future. You have begun to take control. Feelings of being frightened and helpless are often as uncomfortable, or more so, than the actual pain in your back.

CHAPTER THREE
CAUSES
OF BACK PAIN

☐

Delineating causes of back pain produces both frustration and apprehension. Literature on the complexities of back anatomy and physiology, when you have the patience to pursue it, demonstrates your back's vulnerability to possible problems but does little to relate the separate entities of structure, cause, diagnosis, and the cure or prognosis for the future. At this point in your practical what-to-do guide, a foundation of basic, relevant information is offered, with diagrams, to assist you in visualizing possible problems and their inter-relationships, giving you as much rationale as possible for your responses. Back pain is not entirely a medical mystery.

Notwithstanding the oft-repeated "once a back patient, always a back patient," back pain is more often one of mechanics than unlucky happenstance. Chances are good that you can prevent relapse and, more important, prevent a problem from occurring in the first place.

Knowing the relevant facts about the geography of your back helps give meaning to the exercises and body positions you will be practicing. Further information on your back and what could go wrong with it, as well as what you might do about it, will be included in the chapter on medical problems and in the Bibliography.

THE PREVENTION IS THE CURE, AND THE CURE IS THE PREVENTION

Is exertion the problem and rest the cure? The problem has long been perceived more or less in this way.

Except for the initial rest period following a fresh new back attack, the prevention and the cure are virtually the same, and whatever the problem, the cure is the same, whether the problem is primarily one of muscles, ligaments, discs, or even bones. Your body does the healing. You provide the treatment.

As possible adjuncts to your treatment there are collars and braces, muscle relaxants and painkillers, traction, spinal manipulation, acupuncture and massage, and surgery, too. Even so, the more extensive the problem the more intense is the ongoing, persistent, day-to-day care directed toward maximizing back fitness.

POSSIBLE CAUSES OF BACK PAIN

Back strain is far and away the most common cause of back pain. A sprain involves a more severe injury. A disc problem is still more severe and may be the culmination of repeated episodes of back strain or postural problems.

With some exceptions, more than likely you will not

know the diagnosis, whether strain, sprain, disc, or something else. Muscle, ligament, nerve, and joint problems often are interrelated. For example, problems with muscles and bones can place stress on discs. Disc problems may affect nerves and muscles. Stress on joints can impinge on discs. Examining the outline of the bigger picture helps to dispel the doubts and confusion and to clarify the issues. Even without a definitive diagnosis, it assists you in tracking your self-help efforts.

The medical director of the Lahey Clinic's Back School prefers to talk about an "irritated focus" of pain rather than a specific cause for most back pain. There is so much overlap of soft tissues and bone that the same pain can be generated by a number of sources, including discs, ligaments, nerves, and muscles. Therefore, after ruling out serious disease, the cause is described as an "irritated focus," with exercise as the best prescription.

BACK STRAINS AND SPRAINS

Most back pain, it is postulated, results from strain or sprain. Muscle strain results when muscles and tendons are stretched beyond their normal capacity. Tissue fluid may collect, producing pressure, and irritation from blood or tissue fluid on nerve endings may cause pain. Surrounding muscle fibers may then contract to splint the area. The spasm spreads to still wider areas as more muscle fibers contract. Strains may take days or weeks to resolve.

Athletic trainers consider the possibility that chronically contracted muscles, as in stress situations or when there is a need to maintain a particular body position such as sitting or standing for prolonged periods of time, may impede blood circulation, thereby inhibiting the removal of waste products of muscle tissues and resulting in pain. It is thought that chronically contracted muscle fibers may become fatigued and damaged, forming bits of scar tissue. Also muscle fibers not regularly both stretched and strengthened will become chronically shortened. Muscles that are not regularly stretched to maintain their flexibility are especially vulnerable to sudden injury.

Back sprain involves a partial or total tearing of a ligament or tendon. Small muscle fibers may also be torn. A sprain, more serious than a strain, requires a longer time to heal because the blood supply of ligaments and tendons is not as rich as that of muscles. Pulling and stretching of the injured area delay recovery, a reason for rest until pain subsides, and a reason always for halting any exercise or body posture that produces pain. Muscle tears require about six weeks to heal. Ligament healing time is approximately three months.

Healing can be slow and uncertain and occurs by the formation of scar tissue. As a result of these injuries, elasticity of tissues can be diminished because scar tissue is not characterized by elasticity.

Tendons are connective fibers that hold bones to muscles. Ligaments are strong elastic bands that are connected to bone and that bind the discs and joints, connecting bone to bone. Ligaments help to support the vertebrae in place. Both ligaments and tendons can be overstretched due to poor posture, poor muscle tone, incorrect body mechanics, and injury from accidents.

THE DISC STORY

Further stress on the structures of the back may pave the way for disc problems. Discs are those cushioning pads between each of the bones in your back, excluding only the five lowest vertebrae, the sacrum, and the coccyx (tailbone). Frequently disc problems are associated with a history of repeated acute strains at the curve of the lower back just above the sacrum, where it arches. This is called the lumbar and sacral junction, or the sacroiliac joint. For some, a disc problem is the first sign of back trouble with no recall of prior pain. Medical tests can help to determine whether one or more discs are involved. Most back pain is not disc-related, but it may be or may become so.

The vertical muscles on either side of the spine holding your back erect are not large or particularly strong for the work they perform. They can be strengthened, however. A weak back continuously stressed, or suddenly stressed (as by a fall), may require only a so-called trivial trauma to produce a disc rupture.

When apparently healthy adults become suddenly disabled after no more than a cough or a sneeze, or a simple bending motion, the state of one's back can take on an unexpected and understandable importance. The situation demands whatever answers can be found. The best prevention is a back care program started long before a disc or any kind of back problem is identified, one designed to include muscle stretching and strengthening, not only the abdominal muscles, but also the neck, chest, back, leg, buttock, and hip muscles combined with correct postural information. This is the broad outline for both the prevention and the cure.

Discs have a rubbery consistency very much like cartilage and act as shock absorbers for the spine. There are twenty-three discs in your back, and they are thickest in your lower back or lumbar region and thinnest in the thoracic or chest area. During childhood the discs have such strength that an impact injury will crack a spinal bone before injuring a disc.

Incorrect posture combined with weak muscles; damaged, overstretched ligaments; and bone problems can all put many pounds of unusual pressure on the discs. Damaged discs can then exert pressure on nerves, causing back muscles to contract into painful spasm. It is difficult to know whether the pain comes from the muscle spasm, which tends to protect the injured area, or from the pressure the injured disc places on a nerve emerging from the spinal cord.

Discs may become flattened, and this may affect the way the spinal bones glide over each other. Discs may protrude between the spinal bones, called herniation, or may rupture, spilling their contents, and if this occurs, they cannot regenerate. This does not mean that no healing takes place. Disc fragments irritating nerve roots may over time be gradually absorbed. Escaped material from a ruptured disc looks like pieces of crabmeat. A herniated disc problem may take longer to resolve than a disc rupture problem.

Before you were born the discs contained blood vessels, but after birth they have no blood supply. It is believed that the changes in pressure on them as you recline, stand, and move stimulate the circulation of tissue fluids that nourish them. In the morning the discs contain the most fluid, and you may even be a bit taller then than later in the day. A suggestion from the American Physical Therapy Association is to avoid shoveling snow early in the morning because many "slipped" discs occur in the morning, presumably because of the extra fluid pressure within them after a night's sleep.

When you arise and move about, the massaging action of the vertebrae eliminates the extra fluid and "stiffness" some people report in the morning. Astronauts, weightless in space, have reported this problem. Of course, you can always do "warm-up" exercises first, but shoveling anything requires a fit back and can be done only at the very end of your back fitness program, and done correctly using body muscles to minimize disc pressure.

The central portion of the disc is semiliquid, and the material has a shiny appearance during youth, but as time passes there are progressive changes which can become evident by the third decade of life. The inner disc material may lose its liquid central portion. The disc may bulge backward. Fissures, or cracks, in the surrounding fibrous tissue may allow some of the disc material to escape; if it is lost, the liquid may be absorbed. If it coagulates, it may compress a nerve root. After a disc ruptures, blood vessels invade the area, tending to heal the defect and absorb the degenerated tissue. Most likely to rupture or protrude (herniate) is the fourth lumbar disc, which may compress the fifth lumbar nerve root. Discs do not "slip" out of place despite the former frequent use of the term "slipped disc." They bulge, usually in the direction of your back, or they rupture. There may also be a disc

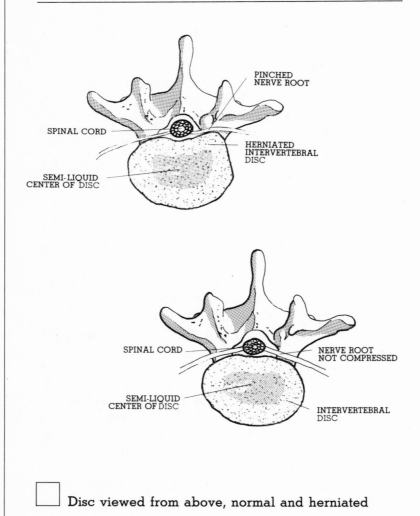

Disc viewed from above, normal and herniated

problem in the neck region, where the cervical discs are located.

This fibrous tissue encircling the central portion of the disc inserts into, or attaches to, the long vertical ligament and then to spinal bones. The posterior longitudinal ligament, the "yellow ligament," is a weak structure, and damage to this ligament can leave a permanently weak-

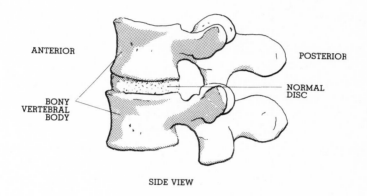

SIDE VIEW

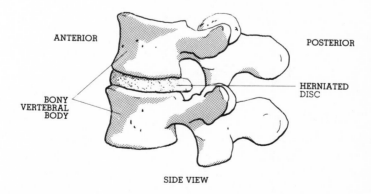

SIDE VIEW

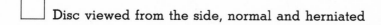
Disc viewed from the side, normal and herniated

ened back. The ligament can tear, weakening it and increasing the likelihood of disc prolapse. Lying just in back of the spinal canal, this ligament is pulled taut when you bend forward from the waist, an activity that subjects this ligament to substantial pressure. There is also an anterior ligament in front of the spine.

When disc material is lost and the space between the vertebrae narrows, the spine may become less stable. The disc space does not narrow immediately to show the rupture on an X-ray film, nor does back pain necessarily accompany disc changes. After a time narrowed disc spaces result in an enlarged bony growth of the vertebrae because the added pressure promotes increased bone formation. Later, arthritic changes may be associated with these bone changes.

Discs may rupture during pregnancy because at this time the joints are relaxed as a result of the release of the pituitary hormone relaxin, therefore increasing the possibility of injury, whether strain, sprain, or disc. Remember, extra abdominal weight increases pressure on the discs. Why? Because it deepens the spine's normal curve as the buttocks push out to compensate for the abdominal weight.

Prolonged confinement to bed, for any reason, increases the risk of having a ruptured disc.

YOUR AGING DISCS

Advancing age tends to be associated with disc changes as discs become firmer and tend to flatten, contributing to loss of height. Loss of bone with advancing age may also contribute to height loss. However, as previously stated, disc changes do not in themselves cause back pain. In fact, the firmer consistency may even be an advantage in regard to potential herniation or rupture problems. Back pain in late middle age or the elderly may be misdiagnosed as disc-related. At this life stage the firmness of the disc material makes it unlikely that the pain is due to a herniated or ruptured disc, a problem associated with younger age groups. It is possible, however, that some of the dried disc tissue may crack or crumble, again not necessarily producing symptoms.

There is no firm information on whether disc changes observed to accompany aging may be at least hastened by long-continued stress or misuse of the back. For example, is the rate of narrowing of disc spaces increased by long-distance running on hard pavement with inadequate cushioning of the feet, or by a gait that produces excessive jarring forces on the spine? What are the results of a lifetime of prolonged sitting, a position placing maximum force on the discs? What are the ways of minimizing disc stress while sitting? We do have answers to the second question.

NERVES AND BACK PAIN

The spinal cord is encased within the bony vertebrae of your back, and from the cord thirty-one pairs of spinal nerves branch out openings in the bones to the rest of your body and up to your brain. Pressure on nerves, whether from discs or impingement of bone, may cause pain, numbness, loss of muscle mass in the legs, and other problems. In the upper back a disc problem may produce numbness in the arms because of pressure on a nerve.

Nerve fibers carry messages to and from the brain. Sensation and pain (sensory) messages are received by the brain, and motor messages are sent from the brain to initiate muscle activity. Sciatic pain is widely heralded as a symptom of back injury because, when a disc is involved, pressure on the sciatic nerve may produce pain that radiates down the legs.

The sciatic nerve is the largest nerve in the body,

extending down the back of your thigh. Because of its position, a herniated disc, a certain type of hip dislocation, or pressure from the uterus during pregnancy may result in sciatic pain.

BACKBONES

The column of separate vertebrae rest one upon the other to form the spine, with the cushioning discs between all but the lower five fused vertebrae. The alignment is a shallow ''s,'' the position you strive to maintain because it places the least stress on bones, discs, muscles, and ligaments. Exaggerating any of these curves as a maintained position, except for brief interludes in positions with reduced gravitational pressure, stresses all the structures of the back.

The newborn spine is formed in the shape of a ''c.'' As the infant begins to raise its head, a curve in the neck appears. As the child begins to stand, a curve in the lower back develops.

There are actually four curves in the spine, including the curve of the neck and the forward curve of the tailbone. The lower back curve, called the lordotic curve, must not be exaggerated into a ''swayback,'' a position that leaves it unstable and vulnerable to injury. Nor should the chest cave in with shoulders dropping forward to exaggerate the forward curve at chest level. And the neck should not be dropped onto the chest, nor shortened and settled back into the shoulders. The back is most protected when the normal, shallow curves are maintained, whether you are walking, sitting, bending, rowing, bicycling, playing tennis, or performing any activity at all.

The winged projections from each vertebra do not impinge on its neighboring bones above and below it. Yet the back can twist from side to side to a moderate

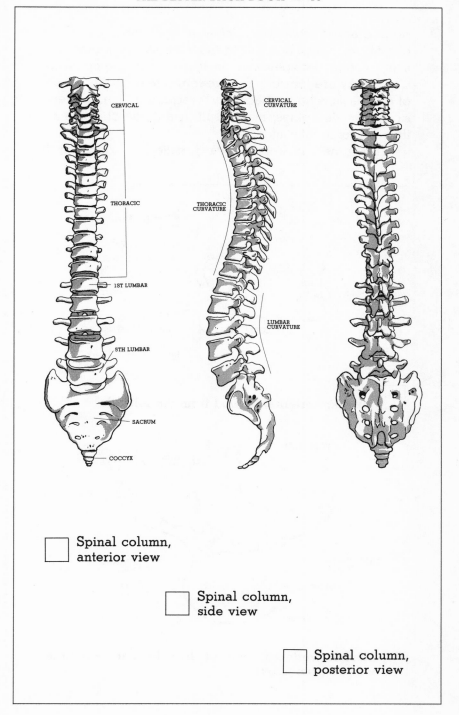

CERVICAL

THORACIC

1ST LUMBAR

5TH LUMBAR

SACRUM

COCCYX

CERVICAL
CURVATURE

THORACIC
CURVATURE

LUMBAR
CURVATURE

☐ Spinal column,
anterior view

☐ Spinal column,
side view

☐ Spinal column,
posterior view

degree at the lower back level and still more so at the chest level. This is because the shape of the vertebrae has some variation depending on the level of the spine in which they are located. The wear and tear on the bones of gymnasts, who do backbends requiring "hyperextension" of their spines, may result in arthritic changes of their backs in later life.

The spine can bend forward, called "flexion," and

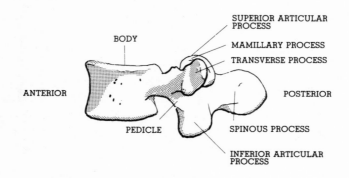

Lumbar vertebra, viewed from the left side

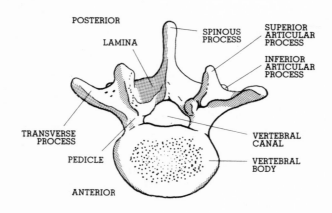

Lumbar vertebra, one of five lumbar vertebrae, viewed from above

backward, called "extension." Each vertebra can angle only slightly, but in aggregate, as each vertebra is brought forward or backward, the back has a wide angle of motion. It can also bend from side to side in a lateral motion. This chain of separate bones is held in alignment by ligaments and supportive muscles. Attached to this important column of bones is the head, which can pivot on the uppermost vertebra called the atlas, the ribs, and the pelvic girdle.

Loss of bone with advancing age, associated with calcium loss and that of other minerals, can result in substantial deterioration of the spine, including the well-known and often very visible "dowager's hump" in the upper back, the exaggerated forward curve in the upper back. If the bones have been weakened by osteoporosis, the discs may even exert an expansive pressure sufficient to indent the vertebrae.

Arthritic changes, "a touch of arthritis," are associated with disc loss and bony changes that may be the result of disc loss, as well as postural defects and occupational risks.

Scoliosis, present to a small degree among many, is a condition in which the spine tends to bend sideways. Scoliosis can put added stress on muscles, ligaments, and discs to increase the risk of back pain.

Another common condition of the spine is sacralization. Those winglike projections on each side of a vertebra may be joined to its neighboring bone on one or both sides, forming an extra joint, usually in the lumbar region, putting strain on the disc during twisting and bending, especially if the joining occurs on only one side of the vertebra. Sacralization occurs during the embryonic life stage. For some occupations, such as truck driving, preemployment physical examinations in the past sometimes included a spinal X ray to rule out this condition. Again, the stronger your back and the greater your understanding of how to use it, the less chance of injury and pain even if sacralization is present.

Vertebrae can be fractured in accidents. Fractures of

the vertebral bones may not show easily on an X ray. One or more cracked vertebrae are not uncommon when sudden or violent pressure is exerted on them, as in a fall or vehicular accident. The possibility exists of accompanying spinal cord injury.

FACET JOINTS: WHAT ARE THEY?

First, what is a joint? There is more than one kind. Bones may be joined by cartilage. Or there may be a hollow part of a bone into which another bone fits (ball and socket), with ligaments holding bones in place and controlling the degree of motion. There are gliding joints where bone slides over bone. Joint dislocation involves derangement of the articulating bones of the joint. Some joints, such as the elbow, have a wide range of motion, unlike those of the back.

A facet is a small, plane surface on a hard body. In the case of your back, it is the flat surface on the vertebra that is the place of union where it meets the same surface of the adjoining vertebra. The facets are the small, flat surfaces on either side of the spinal bones that you can feel when you move your hands along the knobby places of your back. Normally each facet glides smoothly on the surface of its neighbors above and below.

Practitioners such as osteopaths and chiropractors focus specific attention on the facet joints, and orthopedic surgeons also recognize the possibility of "facet joint syndrome." Evidence on X ray may be lacking, and even surgery may not elicit definitive information for diagnosis. Manipulation of the spine may be done with the goal of realigning the spinal vertebrae to relieve pain, including pain from muscle spasm. The muscle spasm may be the result of stress on ligaments and joints deriving from misaligned facets.

Muscle or nerve pain, it is hypothesized, may result from misalignment, and disc damage could also occur. Controversy continues as to how much of a role facet joints play in back pain, but the possibility exists. It is known that facet joints can become worn, whether through osteoporosis; time; misuse of the back, as in chronic back arching; or long-forgotten falls or accidents. And ligaments holding the joints in alignment may become overstretched or torn. An injury can cause dislocation. A damaged disc, making the spine less stable, may increase possibilities of misalignment.

Use of the "hanging" therapies is an attempt to address this problem of alignment, as back sufferers hang from bars or tree branches or have traction therapy. Sudden or excessive pressures on muscles or joints and subsequent injury may result from hanging, whether the body remains upright or is inverted. (See Chapter Eleven for further discussion.)

MORE ON MUSCLES

A muscle is an organ that, by contracting, allows motion of various parts of your body. The smooth muscles of your heart, bladder, stomach, and other internal organs are not under your direct voluntary control, although their contractility can be altered by your emotions—for example, by a rapid heart rate. The striated, or striped, muscles you do control are divided into bundles separated by connective tissue, and as described previously, are attached by tendon to the bones. Nerve impulses cause them to contract.

Muscle cell production halts shortly before birth. You can enlarge your muscle mass, but not the number of individual fibers, by increasing the work load you place on muscles, the result being increased thickness of muscle fibers and increased strength. Individual muscle cells are cylindrical and may be twelve inches long. You cannot strengthen tendons and ligaments. You can only protect them from injury, through increased muscle strengthening and proper body mechanics. If muscles are adequately strong and flexible, you may be able to make a number of errors in the ways you bend and lift without obvious damage to your back.

Muscle tissue constitutes nearly half of your body weight. Muscles are usually in a state of continuous activity, set into motion by nerve impulses. Muscles move venous blood back to the heart, permit you to breathe, and, by contracting, produce body heat. They can be stretched by the action of opposing muscles, and they can contract.

Muscle fibers can be torn if sudden, excessive, or inappropriate loads are placed on muscles unprepared for this stress, either through lack of strength, or, because they have not been stretched, lack of needed flexibility.

Your back is held in alignment and protected by many muscles in addition to the relatively small spinal muscles. The abdominals, which are of prime importance, reach all the way from the sternum in the chest to the pubic bone at the base of your abdomen. There are layers of abdominal muscle tissue, some of which is angled to the side in a crisscross fashion, as well as the vertical muscle tissue. Upper back, shoulder, side, thigh, neck, buttock, knee, calf, and foot muscles are also involved in protecting your back, directly or indirectly. Your muscles both activate your back and limit its range of motion to help prevent injury.

Muscles work in balance with opposing muscles. As one set is being flexed, the opposing set is being stretched. Overdevelopment of one set of muscles may affect postural alignment and cause back pain. For example, tightly contracted upper thigh muscles (quadriceps) and weak hamstring muscles at the back of the thigh may result in an overly straightened or hyperextended knee joint. In this case the knee is more vulnerable to potential injury, and possibly the back as well, because hyperextended knees are associated with swayback.

A sedentary life-style, as in office work where extensive sitting is required, has been mentioned as being a major risk factor for back pain. Interestingly, it has even been found that more than one episode of sprained ankle is a predictor of future back problems. Again, both are indicators of neglected muscle conditioning.

Severely low body weight is associated with back pain, even if an active exercise program is part of the picture. In an eating disorder known as anorexia nervosa, in which intake of calories and nutrients is severely restricted, not only fat and muscle but even bone may be lost. Lack of muscle tissue may be a reason that anorexia nervosa appears, at times, to be associated with back problems. For instance, lack of muscle tissue in the buttocks may permit unusual pressure on the sciatic nerve, causing pain in the lower back and legs.

UPPER BACK PROBLEMS

Pain in the upper back can be severe, and it can be chronic. Many of the same factors operate in neck and shoulder pain as in the lower back. It is frequently associated with prolonged sitting at a desk or video display terminal and is increased by tension and postural factors. There may have been a whiplash injury. Pain may occur in the neck or shoulders, or between the shoulder blades. Numbness of the arms is associated with disc injury. Muscle strain occurs in the upper back as in the lower back, although the complaint is less frequent and often, but not necessarily, less disabling. Again, the self-help approach is postural change, and muscle stretching and strengthening exercises, with the possibility, as in lower back pain, of the need for medical intervention.

THE ROLE OF STRESS

It is usually meaningless to ascribe back pain to the ill-defined, catchall category of stress, which leaves people not knowing how to respond. It is possible that, even after belatedly receiving information on back protection and strengthening, the pressures of time and various responsibilities may result in chronically tight, shortened muscles. The stress of time pressures may lead to reduced attention to proper bending and lifting techniques, lessened allocation of time for appropriate exercise, and less attention to necessary changes of body position. When one is distracted by other concerns, early pain signals may be ignored. It is hypothesized that those who are considered to be perfectionists may have more risk of back pain.

RISKY BUSINESS

Anyone who performs a specific, repetitive task over a prolonged period of time appears to be especially vulnerable to back pain. The occupation might be working at a drafting table, playing the cello, standing behind a counter, driving a car or truck, or any one of a myriad of other tasks that require repetitive use of the same muscles and body position. In these situations sustained tension of certain muscle groups is involved. According to one study, people who spend at least half of their job time driving a motor vehicle are three times more likely than the average worker to have a herniated disc. Bus drivers were found to have more back problems than their peripatetic fare collectors on the same vehicle.

Habitual bending forward from your waist to weed

your garden, or twisting as you bend forward to lift your child over the edge of a crib can be very risky. Pushing a vacuum cleaner for prolonged periods of time can be an invitation to back pain. Doing sit-up exercises with straight knees can damage your back. Touching your toes without bending your knees puts your back at risk. Push-ups with straight knees can bring on back pain. The reasons for all of the above will become clear.

Not wearing seat belts and shoulder harnesses leaves you vulnerable to strain, sprain, and disc injury; fractured vertebrae; facet joint misalignment; nerve and spinal cord injury and to other injuries, not related to your back.

CHAPTER FOUR
GETTING MOVING

This chapter is directed especially to those who are experiencing current back pain or who are recovering from an acute back attack. Some people with mild back strain but who are in moderately good physical condition are pain-free within two or three days. Others may require a longer time, but feel fine as long as they do not stand or sit for "too long."

The *New England Journal of Medicine* article cited in the Bibliography documents a lack of increased benefit with prolonged bed rest. The study suggests no difference in outcome between a group of patients for whom two days of bed rest were prescribed and a group for whom seven days of bed rest were prescribed except for increased absenteeism from work in the latter group. Two hundred patients without neurologic symptoms or other illness were studied, and a three-month follow-up examination was done.

But judgment is required in making individual decisions about optimum balance between rest and exercise. Sometimes people start to become active by performing an activity such as carrying the laundry, raking the garden, or taking the bus to the office. Then they backtrack as they experience pain and do less. Being up and active is not the same as following a sequential, graded program of exercise. It may be true that patients tend to get better no matter what they do. In a sense, hearing this may be reassuring, but it does not address the problem of relapse.

Before resuming "normal activities," consider the benefits and risks of bed rest. Then do the following: First, ice a new or suspected injury. Second, learn muscle relaxation techniques. Third, try moist heat if you wish. Fourth, carefully stretch out your lower back muscles that may be in spasm regardless of the primary cause of back pain. Fifth, start the Level One back exercises performed in the flat position and do not stress your back.

No sooner do you get settled into bed rest for your "enforced vacation" than you will find yourself thinking about when, and especially how, you will again begin to live a normal life up on your feet.

At first any thought of activity may tend to give you pause. Sometimes the pain is intermittent, even disappearing entirely, especially while you lie down. Will getting up cause your pain to return? Will you hurt yourself unknowingly? If you do hurt yourself, will you know if the injury may not be apparent immediately? The same fears may recur later when you consider starting to learn a new sport such as tennis, golf, basketball, or horseback riding. Information is remarkably lacking, but for the majority of backaches, an occasional walk around the house is considered beneficial, adding further activity slowly. If getting up causes or increases your pain, the advice is to remain flat, not propped. Sometimes a back injury or disc problem does not permit you to walk.

Start Level One exercises before you do any significant amount of walking. By doing so, you can avoid the compression effect of gravity that results when you assume the standing position.

These first bed exercises help to begin the process of stretching your back muscles and shortening your abdominal muscles. Your time in bed may be lessened by becoming proficient in the Level One exercises. Even though weeks or months are required for complete healing, the exercises help to increase your "up time" before your back muscles start to spasm, whether the spasm results from injury to muscles, ligaments, or discs, or all of these.

Pain is a subjective sensation not easily documented by medical tests. Often it seems to come and go for no logical reason, apparently independent of what you do or do not do. Sometimes you think you can walk across the parking lot, but partway across the lot your back almost literally gives out as you feel a sudden spasm of pain. You cannot predict, especially at first, but neither can anyone else, even the experts. After a while you can expect to gain a measure of understanding of what your body can do. The general rule is always to do nothing that causes or increases pain.

BED REST: THE PROS

There are reasons that rest continues to be the first line of defense in treating back pain. Why? Because pain is usually reduced or eliminated in the horizontal position, presumably because of removal of the strain of gravity and body weight, therefore allowing muscles in spasm to relax. With less pressure on the back structures, healing can begin. If there is swelling of tissues or inflammation, this can subside. The restricted movement involved in bed rest reduces the risk of back spasm and maladaptive body mechanics such as in twisting motions. Lifting and incorrect ways of sitting are eliminated.

BED REST: THE CONS

But bed rest by itself cannot be depended upon as the major or the sole solution to your back attack. After only a few days it has major effects on your whole body, including weakening the very muscles you need to hold yourself erect. Within ten days you may actually lose up to a third of your thigh muscle strength! Therefore, no matter how long you must remain in bed, you should begin conditioning your body even, as stated above, in those first days.

Older people in particular must be discouraged from relying on bed rest if their backs hurt. For them almost any bed rest can be detrimental at worst and ineffective at best, and it should be attempted only if the clinician supplies an adequate reason; an inflammatory process of some sort might require rest. Without a compelling reason, elderly people cannot afford to lose muscle strength and flexibility.

Currently there are concerns about calcium loss from bones without the weight-bearing activities of normal living. Progressive bone loss begins in the midthirties, especially among women. Weight-bearing exercise such as walking, running, pulling, and lifting has been found to be a factor in retarding the rate of bone loss, which, in later years, can result in back problems and bone fractures. A few days of bed rest or weightlessness, as in space travel, result in measurable loss of calcium from bones.

Also, the circulation of your blood is diminished by bed rest. So knowing that bed rest is not the panacea it was once thought to be, you should try to do all you can to expedite your progress by increasing your pain-free-on-your-feet-time as rapidly as possible.

FIRST DAYS

When you change position, as you probably will at intervals, from side to back, or back to side, or from side to side, how you do it may make a difference. Plan your move rather than jerking yourself into position.

Get the covers, if any, out of the way. Move slowly, keeping your body as much aligned as possible. When switching sides, lead with your bent knees and follow with your shoulders while trying to prevent your body from twisting. Even if you are not currently having a back attack, it is wise to slow down any tendency to make sudden, uncontrolled moves. Motions should be smooth.

Exercise physiologists, aerobics instructors, and relaxation classes now move in the direction of childbirth preparation classes in combining breathing techniques with tension and release of muscles. Always the emphasis is on "don't hold your breath." Why? Two reasons are: (1) You tense muscles that should be involved in the activity and (2) you interrupt oxygen intake at a time when you may need more, not less, oxygen. Exercise classes and exercise videotapes remind you constantly, "breathe," "don't hold your breath."

You should breathe diaphragmatically, which means that you should expand your waist and abdomen as you inhale, not your ribs and chest. Inhale over a count of about five seconds, or whatever is comfortable for you, and exhale in a sighing breath, also about five seconds in length, through pursed lips so you can hear the sound. You will feel your body relax because this breath acts to release tension. You are always encouraged to perform any exercise, or motion, on the exhalation breath. Merely changing position in bed may not require that you breathe in any particular way, but here is an opportunity to practice. Later, when you plan to move your picnic table, it may become much more important.

BALANCING ACT

From the beginning, recovery involves a number of factors that, at first glance, may appear to be in opposition. You learn muscle relaxation and stress reduction. At the same time, muscle strengthening begins to be a significant part of your daily life. Muscles need also to be stretched regularly to prevent back pain. The ways you use your body, "body mechanics," must be addressed, even the way you get out of bed. For example, do you jerk yourself to a sitting position, or do you, as pregnant women have been taught for years, first roll to your side and use your hands and shoulders to raise your body from the bed as you swing your bent knees over the side?

How do you know how to balance these apparently opposing factors? How much of each and when? Does this balance change as you progress through the recovery program? How do you know how fast you can progress through the increased levels of activity? Specific "what to do when" information has long been notably lacking, and most back programs have limited their exercises to the standard few. The integration of relaxation, stress management, body mechanics, muscle strengthening, muscle stretching, and "what to do when" information has been generally unavailable.

Already stated is the remarkable fact that the prevention and the cure of back pain are virtually the same whatever its cause. Even with the answers far from complete, these pages will assist in taking you a few steps farther along the route to a faster and more complete recovery as well as in showing you how to prevent becoming enmeshed in back problems in the first place.

STRETCHING OUT YOUR BACK

While you concentrate on your back muscles, sore or not, consciously let go of the muscles of your back and relax them "outward" as you lie on your side, increasing the outward curve of your back. Placing a heating pad, or better, a hot water bottle against your back may enhance your ability to release these muscles as you relax against the warmth. Take in a deep, slow breath and release it, focusing on letting go of muscle tension as you exhale. Note that stretching means curving, not straightening or arching your back.

Pause a bit. Now try, very slowly, to bring your knees up toward your chest. Your neck is inclined somewhat forward and your back curves outward at the waist. If your neck were inclined backward instead, your back muscles would not be able to relax. Normally you would expect to have no difficulty in bringing your knees close to your chest with your ankles tucked against your thighs. If your back is stiff, move only inches at a time before pausing and once again relaxing. When you feel any significant pull, or if this causes increased pain, stop and straighten out your body enough to relieve the discomfort. Always aim to avoid pain. Rest at this point. As you repeat this back stretching position several times a day you should see progress. Maggie Lettvin (see Bibliography) has identified this "fetal" position as the first that one should assume whenever back pain strikes. Although it is possible to bring your knees to your chest with your back arched, rather than being curved outward, it should be avoided.

This side-lying back stretch, when later done on your feet, is actually a squat without the compressive gravitational effects on your back muscles, ligaments, and discs and without the need to maintain your balance. Until you have the flexibility to assume this position you will not be able to begin to consider lifting anything because lifting requires bending your knees and lowering yourself to whatever you wish to lift. Yet there are those who are surprised to find that they are expected to be able to draw their knees to their chests. They have scarcely thought about squatting down on their heels since they were children, and it is not even possible when wearing narrow skirts or tight pants. The results are tight backs and weak thighs. Can back pain be far behind?

As you practice in bed you will be able to draw your knees farther toward your chin. You will be able to identify contracted back muscles and tight hamstring muscles that go from the buttocks down the back of the thigh. You can identify lack of flexibility of your knee joints. Yes, knees, too, can be involved in back pain. This exercise is an important step toward stretching muscles particularly associated with backache. The first was lying in bed with your knees raised.

If you have a new, fresh back injury, you may find that you have to wait before doing this exercise. In the meantime, simply rest on your side with flexed knees, your back curved slightly outward, and remain as relaxed as you can manage.

RELAXATION RESPONSE

The relaxation response is taught in many health promotion classes for possible relief of headaches, high blood pressure, and stress management. It also belongs in a take-care-of-your-back program.

The relaxation response first entered medicine's mainstream by way of Herbert Benson, M.D. Long before Benson's book (see Bibliography), Edmund Jacobsen, a physiologist, had taught progressive muscle relaxation as a means of reducing pain. Childbirth classes have utilized muscle relaxation since the 1940s to reduce the pain of labor, which involves periodic contraction of the involuntary uterine muscle. The relaxation response can be adapted in a variety of ways. Its primary purpose in a back care program is to release tight muscles and help you think before you move.

It is known that better muscle relaxation can be obtained by stretching muscles before relaxing them instead of in tightening them before releasing them. However, stretching the various parts of the body requires knowledge, and will be included in the chapter on Level Three exercises. As you stretch one muscle group you contract the opposing muscle group. Both tightening and releasing muscles aid muscle tone and blood circulation in addition to enhancing relaxation. The following sequence is suggested:

1. Remain quiet in as comfortable a position as possible, on your side with knees bent or on your back with raised knees. Be sure that you are warm enough so that you can relax. A cold room can produce obvious muscle tension in the form of shivering, but being even slightly cool increases muscle tension.

2. Slowly tighten one fist over a time period of several seconds.

3. Slowly release the tension over a time period of several seconds while exhaling. Note that this is the exception to contracting muscles while exhaling.

4. Do the same with the other fist.

5. Point your heel while slowly tensing the foot and leg muscles. By pointing the heel, not the toe, your calf muscle is stretched.

6. Exhale while releasing slowly, in a controlled manner, the tension in that foot and leg.

7. Do the same with the other heel.

8. Close your eyes and press firmly with your fingers around the bony orbits of your eyes.

9. Inhale, then exhale, consciously letting go of all the muscles in your face.

10. Slowly draw in your abdominal muscles, but stop if you find your back muscles also tensing or hurting. Release them after a few seconds.

12. Breathe regularly, slowly, and deeply for several minutes while maintaining as complete muscle relaxation as possible throughout your body.

13. Try a visualization technique, such as picturing yourself lounging on a tropical beach seeing blue water, green mountains, islands, whatever you prefer. Perhaps you will choose to float in a balloon over an endless forest.

14. Unaccustomed as you may be, adopt a passive attitude, permitting relaxation to occur at its own pace. When distracting thoughts or images occur, try to ignore them and repeat the word "one" silently to yourself. Continue the regular, slow, deep breathing pattern.

When you "come back to the real world" do so slowly, starting with half-opened, unfocused eyes. Needless to say, do not use an alarm clock, or have an alarm-clock mind-set. Many people in their daily lives make a point of practicing relaxation for a time or two each day for ten or twenty minutes, not because they have any particular medical problem but just because they feel better when they do.

While you remain in a somewhat reflective mood you could note that had you had a back pain problem a generation ago your doctor might have tried to help you by taping up your back with adhesive tape in an attempt to prevent more injury and to try to support your back. History does not record the pain involved in removing those wide bands of adhesive tape! Today corsetry and back braces are available, to be used only if a need is identified in consultation with one's medical care provider. For many this does not help. Issues of muscle weakness and lack of flexibility are not addressed, and problems with life-style do not go away.

Backache sufferers do, however, often find that a wide belt fastened firmly around the lower waist and upper hip area may allow them to remain up on their feet for a

longer time before their back muscles again go into painful spasm. Those whose physical conditioning program
includes lifting weights, and who have no back pain,
often use a wide leather belt to help avoid injuring their
lower backs as they lift.

CHAPTER FIVE

WHAT NEXT?
LEVEL ONE
BACK EXERCISES

L ocal irritation to joints and nerves subsides gradually and at an uncertain pace. The ratio between the time you are up and the time you are horizontal depends on your pain. When pain occurs you must get off your feet until it resolves. Even if you improve enormously, you may find yourself with an unexpected backache. You cannot allow pain to continue.

Lie down for five to twenty minutes, as you require. A favorite way to relieve pain is to lie on a carpeted floor with thighs at right angles to your back and your legs resting on a chair seat so that they are parallel with your back and the floor.

The amount of pain-free time that you can be up is a measure of your progress in healing and muscle strengthening. As you increase the frequency and challenge of back strengthening exercises, and with the passage of time, pain episodes become more infrequent.

The suggested exercises and activities have been divided into levels of challenge to provide a guide for logical progression in which to practice them. Your back problem may be mild. You may have no current symptoms at all and feel yourself to be generally physically fit, or, at the other end of the spectrum, you may be recovering from an acute, disabling back attack.

In either case, because Level One exercises are fundamental to back health, start at this level. Later you may include these as warm-up exercises to prepare for other physical activity. Also, you should do a series of repetitions at least two or three times a week as a general preventive program.

If your back is still sore, however, try them slowly and carefully a couple of times a day, depending on what you determine is helpful for you if you have had a chronic back problem or have just had a back attack. You may want to consult with your physician for an opinion.

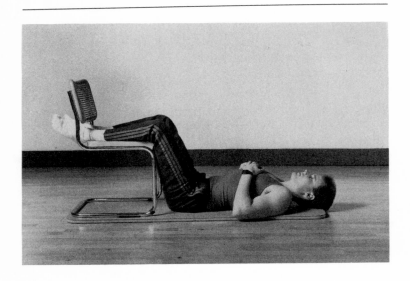

☐ Level One. Position to Relieve Back Pain

The number of repetitions of each and the speed at which you do them will depend on your level of fitness and what your back seems to need. There is no point in suggesting twenty bent-knee sit-ups to someone who cannot, even once, peel himself or herself off the floor.

At the end of this book a back health maintenance program will be suggested. Some people prefer one exercise over another, both offering the same or similar benefits.

WHY EXERCISE? REMEMBERING WHAT YOU KNOW

There are those who rest awhile, stagger to their feet, do a few pelvic tilts, and soak in the health club whirlpool, feeling that the worst is over and hoping for the best. For a while they do an exercise or two, but as they return to normal life their diligent attention to a regimen diminishes and disappears with the pain. It is all a bad memory, now happily behind them.

The lack of compliance in regard to exercise has induced many health care practitioners to feel that their words are wasted when they tell patients that all is not well just because the pain has subsided, that they are in effect sitting on a time bomb of a possible back attack that may at some uncertain time explode, interrupting their daily lives once more. When this does occur the temptation, once again, for patient and practitioner is to depend for the solution on a few days of rest. Prevention for the future is all but ignored.

You may continue to wonder why now, of all times, when you are practically an invalid, you must start an exercise program, especially if you do not know how your back was injured and cannot lift even a cafeteria tray. After reading Chapter Three, on the causes of back pain and how quickly muscle mass declines with inactivity, you know one of the whys.

What if you decide to do no exercises at all? What if you simply rest as the pain requires and nothing else? Situations differ, but the chances are that the pain will subside, but not as fast, nor will the recovery, as indicated above, be as complete. You will find yourself making a point of not stressing your back and, with good reason, fearing that the pain will return. All is not well just because you have no current pain.

Exercise can be viewed in a variety of ways. You may have perceived it as a way to develop skill in a competitive sport, to relieve stress, or as a tiresome chore. Exercise has long had an association with health, and ever since President Kennedy's Council on Fitness, knowledge of and interest in exercise have grown year by year. While behavior change in the school-age population has lagged, the adult population, including men and women sixty and beyond, has seen the proliferation of exercise clothes, health clubs, corporate fitness programs, jogging trails, and community-based fitness classes. Back schools offering two or three sessions on back exercises are sprouting in hospitals and community centers.

The word "aerobics," first publicized by Kenneth Cooper, M.D., more than fifteen years ago, is now in common use. Aerobic exercise increases the strength of your heart muscle, and the efficiency of your cardiovascular system in general, as well as acting to lower your blood pressure and reduce the level of your blood fats and cholesterol, especially the low-density lipoprotein known as the "bad cholesterol." The resultant changes in exercise and diet appear, according to the American Heart Association, to be related to the decreased incidence of heart attacks in the United States.

In light of the importance of aerobic exercise, it is disappointing for many to recognize that aerobic fitness cannot be maintained at the customary level while in the midst of an episode of back pain. Any repetitive activity you might try to increase your heart rate will inevitably lead to tightening and stressing your back muscles. Your back is that important. If you are currently zeroing in on coping with back pain, your level of aerobic fitness will begin to decline within days of interrupting aerobic exercise, but as you become more active, there are ways of helping yourself. Walking and swimming, for most people, can be started fairly soon. Both can offer aerobic benefit.

Exercise, even if not aerobic, burns calories to help maintain normal weight. In addition, it has been found to relieve stress and to be an antidote to depression, due to changes in body chemistry and taking an active approach to resolving a problem, in this case back pain.

A WORD ON BACK EXERCISES

Back exercises done in bed or on a foam mat often appear less burdensome than what many envision as exercise. This is a plus. At the same time they may appear so deceptively mild and nonstrenuous that the need for doing them regularly, for the rest of one's life, seems less compelling than it is. Also, it is normal to question whether simple exercises are being done correctly or that they are doing any good. Few back sufferers have the opportunity to have someone coach them through a comprehensive and understandable program all the way from acute back attack to total back fitness.

Back sufferers often have genuine doubts about exercise as either a preventive measure or as an antidote for back pain. If one has an injury, will exercise really help? In the minds of many, the connection between injury and rest remains strong.

Back exercises, involving both muscle strengthening and stretching, provide positive feedback in terms of reduced pain, reduced probability of recurrence, and measurable increase in muscle strength. Many experience the less visible satisfaction of feeling more in tune with their body and of having more control over it. If you currently have back pain, the "in tune with" and "control over" may not, at the moment, appear either relevant or comprehensible.

"TWENTY QUESTIONS"

Questions and apparent contradictions on how to take care of your back abound in back care classes. Group members often push persistently, and often without success, for clarification.

1. Swimming is described as a most desirable exercise for back patients, yet I am told that my back should not be arched, that the curve of the back should instead be flattened. At what point in my recovery should I start to swim, and what swimming stroke should I use?

2. I am informed that it is important that I stretch my hamstring muscles, but I am discouraged from sitting and from bending forward to touch my toes. How do I reconcile these apparently opposite instructions?

3. I am told that it is important to rest my back, but at the same time I am informed that exercise is the key to recovery. How do I know when and how much of each I should incorporate into my daily program?

4. When can I start lifting packages, groceries, children? When can I lift weights? How will I know how much weight I can carry and for how long?

5. When, if ever, can I resume sleeping on my stomach? Is that the cause of my back pain?

6. I know that the saying "no pain, no gain" has fallen out of favor in all the literature on backache, aerobic exercise, and athletic programs. Do I exercise to the point of pain? I also know that pain may not be evident for as much as several hours after injury. How will I know how much activity I can manage if I do not get immediate feedback from my body?

7. I have heard that strong abdominal muscles are important, but is this the whole story to back care? Just what do the exercises accomplish?

8. How often, how long and at what pace are the exercises done?

9. How many of the exercises need to be done regularly? Are some more important than others?

10. When can I spend part of the day sitting up or going out for a ride in the car? I am told I can return to work, but I am told to avoid riding in a car.

11. I hear that I must not lean forward, yet I must not arch my back so that I lean backward. I must not throw my shoulders back in the so-called military posture, and I must not hold my back stiffly. So just what do I do so I do not move as if I were walking on eggs?

12. As a health club member, what do I need to know about exercise equipment? Will it help my back, or will it injure my back? How do I know when and how to use it to aid in recovery and to help prevent possible back pain in the future?

You may think of other questions, and they may even add up to twenty!

FIRST EXERCISE

SIDE-LYING SQUAT WITH TIGHTENED ABDOMINALS

You have already practiced this position while doing the relaxation response, and stretching out your back to help relieve pain. Do it on your bed or an exercise mat.

Draw your abdominal muscles in tight, another step toward strengthening muscles involved in supporting your back and, in combination with stretched back and hamstring muscles, achieving the famous "pelvic tilt" that will forevermore be your bulwark against future back injury.

As you do this exercise, the lordotic curve in your lower back is reduced to open the posterior, or back, disc spaces of your spine. Later you can do this on your feet, but balance and the effects of gravity are involved, and muscles of your back, buttocks, and hamstrings must first have maximum stretch. Doing this on your feet before you are ready tends to cause injury and pain. On your side you can do a gentle, persistent, and controlled muscle stretch. Do not twist as you do this. Also in this position you can use heat or gentle massage if you wish. Sometimes you can feel which part of your back is sore if you press firmly with your hand; it can be reassuring to discover just where the pain is. Usually it is muscle pain, but remember that muscle spasm is often associated with back pain, whatever its cause.

Place your hands in front of, not behind, your knees, and use your hands to guide your progress in pulling up your knees. Some back programs direct you to place your hands behind your knees. The difference is that if your hands are behind your knees, you may place more pull or stretch on your back than you intended. On the other hand, if you have previously injured one or both knees, placing your hands in front of your knees may put excessive pressure on your knee joints. Stop when you feel significant tightness and before the point of pain. Move slowly. Attempting to hurry may result in defensive muscle tightening. Later you can be slightly more venturesome.

First, take in a deep, satisfying breath, and as you slowly exhale, draw in and tighten your abdomen as much as you possibly can. Move your knees still closer to your chin as you lie with your shoulders and head curled into a "C" position. Do not hold your breath. Maintain this position of maximum abdominal muscle contraction for six to ten seconds. Rest for ten to fifteen seconds before you repeat. Try this exercise at intervals several times each day.

If pressure on the sciatic nerve produces pain when you draw the leg up beyond a certain point, probably in one leg only, you can draw up the other leg. Also periodically attempt to pull the leg that bothers you up to the point of discomfort or pain. Usually that soreness is in the buttock and goes down the back of your leg. The expectation is that the pain in the affected leg will tend to subside. If you have sciatic pain, stay in touch with your doctor.

SECOND EXERCISE

RAISED KNEE PELVIC TILT ON YOUR BACK

Lie on your back with knees raised and feet flat. Press your waist and lower back against a firm surface. Inhale deeply and, as you exhale, slowly, over a count of about six seconds, draw in your abdominal muscles to their maximum, pressing your waist still farther onto the mattress or floor mat. Keep your arms, neck, and shoulders relaxed.

The same exercise can be done with your knees resting on plump pillows. Inhale as you gradually release your contracted abdominals. Pause, rest a few seconds or longer, and repeat. As before, you are reducing the lordotic curve in your lower back, strengthening your abdominals, and, to an extent (but not as much as in the first exercise), stretching your back muscles.

This exercise is important in protecting your back. Yet it will not stress your back, and it is unlikely to produce pain if your back muscles can stretch even slightly. Later, when your back feels tired or achey, this exercise can be used to relieve pain.

THIRD EXERCISE

RAISED KNEE PELVIC TILT ON YOUR BACK WITH CONTRACTED BUTTOCKS

Do the above exercise exactly the same way, but as you tighten your abdomen, also tighten your seat muscles. They need strengthening, too. Some people who have acute back pain find that contracting muscles of the buttocks hurts their backs. If this is the case, wait, and try again later.

Tightening the buttocks increases the effectiveness of the second exercise. However, in a new back attack, or if there is sciatic pain or a disc problem, tightening muscles of the buttocks can sometimes cause pain.

FOURTH EXERCISE

HEAD RAISES

Lie on your back with knees raised. Place the palm of your hands, with fingers touching, across your midsection. Press firmly against your navel to support your abdominal muscles. Inhale, and, as you exhale through pursed lips, contract your abdominal muscles and raise your head up off the bed or exercise mat. Let your head fall back down. Do not jerk your head off the floor. Do the motion smoothly. Many people do not support the abdomen, and as they raise their heads their abdomens rise also. Do not allow this to happen.

Now raise your head without supporting the vertical abdominal muscles (the recti) with your hands. At the level of your navel, press firmly with your fingertips to search for the space between the muscles. A space of an inch or so is normal. If the space is wide, do your best to reduce it by doing head raises while pressing the muscles together with your hands. With your head on the bed you cannot feel the space. It becomes apparent only when you raise your head. The space disappears when you drop your head. Especially after pregnancy, it is essential to check for separation of the recti muscles.

Elizabeth Noble, physical therapist and childbirth educator, has described and stressed the importance of these vertical abdominal muscles and the need to check them. As she states, regarding sit-ups and curl-ups, it makes no sense to ask your abdominal muscles to raise your shoulders off the floor if they cannot stay parallel with only the weight of your head!

And if you do try to raise your shoulders, or if you arch your back, or if you hold your breath, you can actually increase the separation of these muscles. So practice tightening your abdominals with only your head raised at first, keeping your back pressed into the bed, and continue to breathe.

FIFTH EXERCISE

PELVIC TILT ALL FOURS

The pelvic tilt all fours exercise, as does the raised knee pelvic tilt on your back exercise (second exercise), strengthens abdominal and stretches lower back muscles. But you can increase the angle of the tilt, and by so doing you can work the muscles of your upper back, arms, and shoulders to some extent, which the second exercise does not.

The all fours position is not necessarily the ideal position for humankind, despite the allegations that the upright position is a major source of back problems. Nevertheless, many back sufferers find the position comfortable. You may find that a modified version of this relieves pain, such as when you are seated at a desk and lean forward in the chair to rest your forearms on the desk. Kneeling may also offer relief. If you have taken childbirth preparation classes, you already know this exercise.

"Make like a square box," placing your knees under your hips and your hands flat on the floor or firm surface with your fingers pointing ahead of you. Like a cat, arch your lower back up toward the ceiling in a long, leisurely stretch. Your abdominal muscles are used to round your back. It should feel good to your back. Hold the position a few seconds, then lower your back to the flat position. Do not, especially if your back is at all vulnerable to pain, let it sag or arch below the flat position. Repeat, slowly, several times. Later in the day try several more repetitions.

Note that this exercise is described as arching your back, just as this activity is described when observing a cat. Normally, when discussing your back the word "arch" means the opposite and is defined as extending the curve in your lower back as you bend backward. "Flex" means rounding your back as you bend forward.

SIXTH EXERCISE

BACK-LYING PELVIC TILT, LEGS EXTENDED

Lie face up, without a pillow, and with your knees drawn up. Press the middle of your back firmly against the bed with your abdominals contracted. Tighten your buttocks and, slowly, slide one leg down until it is straight. Draw it back to a flexed position and do the same with the other leg, always maintaining your pelvic tilt. Do not hold your breath.

Now, starting with flexed knees, slowly slide both heels down to straighten your legs. If your waist starts to leave the bed as you begin to lose the essential pelvic tilt, halt your heel slide at that point, and try again later. Do this several times a day, holding the position for several seconds at a time. As you practice, you will become aware of increasing muscle strength.

As an added benefit, stretch your arms up straight over your head so your entire body is stretched out straight, your pelvis tilted as a result of the contraction of your seat and abdominal muscles. Stretch your calf muscles by pointing your toes toward the ceiling.

Remember to breathe diaphragmatically, as de-

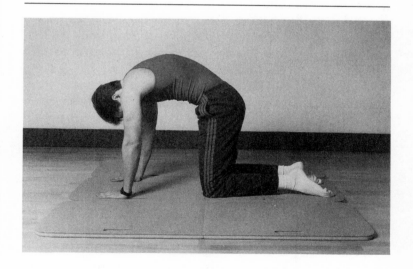

□ Level One. Pelvic Tilt on All Fours

scribed in Chapter Three. Do not breathe by heaving your chest shallowly and irregularly. Contract your muscles on the exhalation breath.

Emphasis on the exhalation breath encourages fuller breathing and discourages bulging muscles as you try to tense them. Maintain a regular breathing rhythm, not tense or jerky. Never hold your breath, because this is associated with inappropriate muscle tension and a temporary rise in blood pressure and can interfere with the smooth performance and benefit of the exercise.

SEVENTH EXERCISE: ON YOUR FEET

THE STANDING PELVIC TILT

The first six exercises prepare you for standing and walking by strengthening the muscles needed for the prolonged upright position and by showing you the pelvic angle providing maximum stability for your back. At first you will find standing and walking more comfortable than sitting. Don't even think of sitting at this point.

Move to a wall and place your feet a few inches from it. Flatten your back against the wall to eliminate as much as possible any space between your back and the wall. Your pelvis is now tilted.

By squeezing your buttocks tightly together, your back is better supported and you strengthen muscles that help to protect your back. Later, if you are standing in a movie line or touring a museum and begin to feel an ache in your back, you may be able to relieve the ache by consciously tilting your pelvis and tightening your buttocks.

Lift your rib cage, but without arching your back, then release your buttock muscles and walk away from the wall.

WARNING WORDS:
THE NO-NOS

Despite the directions on a few exercise sheets you may acquire, do not do the following:

1. Do not do bend over to touch your toes with straight knees, now or later.

2. Do not do straight-leg raises.

3. As you may know, do not do straight-leg sit-ups, now or in the future.

4. Do not do straight-leg push-ups.

CHAPTER SIX

ON YOUR WAY:
LEVEL TWO
BACK EXERCISES

☐

One man, after rupturing a disc in his back while traveling in Europe, reports standing in the airplane all the way from London to the United States, thereby illustrating the preference most back sufferers have when faced with the choice of sitting or standing. When you sit, the whole weight of your body rests on your lower back. When you stand, your legs take some of the pressure and there is no stretching force on possibly tight hamstring muscles. Walking is easier still on your back than standing, as forces on the back are continually shifting rather than being sustained. Therefore, one finds those recovering from back problems often standing or walking about their offices, even at meetings. When they do sit, they get up often. Doing this can help prevent back pain as well as relieve it.

THE "AMATEUR ICE SKATER" STANCE

Back exercises developed by Williams (see Bibliography) focused firmly on the concept of the pelvic tilt, and this emphasis remains at the core of back exercise programs. The pelvic tilt in daily life protects your back as you drive, cook, walk, or swing a golf club. The back is to be flexed, not extended. But as time passes there will be benefit to extending, if not hyperextending, your back for brief periods of time, as found by McKenzie (see Bibliography). Back muscles must be strengthened as well as stretched. For an optimally fit back one of the goals is a flexible spine. A rigidly held spine is associated with aging. Therefore, exercises for a modified back arch will be included among Level Three exercises.

The combined fear of hurting one's back, possible upper body muscle weakness, and the encouragement to maintain the pelvic tilt can result in a round-shouldered stance with a bend at the waist so that the waist is rounded outward. You see this standing position when people learn to skate, when they walk with a cane, brush their teeth, or stand over a kitchen sink. To avoid the swayed back, they exaggerate the tilt. General weakness of muscles supporting the rib cage can encourage this "C" position. Certain activities such as pushing a lawn mower or vacuum cleaner can encourage this stance.

This position is hard on your back because of the strain it places on back muscles, the discs and the ligaments that help bind and support the structures of the lower back. If your knees are slightly flexed, your back has some protection. Even in the horizontal position, do not fold yourself at the waist with your legs straight. It can be confusing. The solution? Do the pelvic tilt, then lift your rib cage to straighten your spine, bring your neck up and out of your shoulders to make a "long neck," and drop your shoulders. Make sure your knees are "unlocked," or you will have difficulty maintaining the pelvic tilt. You are now ready to stride forth.

FIRST EXERCISE

KNEE-TO-CHEST LOWER-BACK STRETCH ON YOUR BACK ONE LEG AT A TIME

Lie on your back with your arms resting at your sides, your head flat or on a small pillow, and your knees raised. Assume the pelvic tilt, by now your watchwords, and wrap both arms around one knee. Draw your knee slowly toward your chest, with no jerking motion, which could cause muscles to tighten defensively against a sudden stretch. Be absolutely certain that your effort to bring the knee farther does not result in arching your back and consequent shortening of your back muscles.

Do the same with the opposite knee, holding the stretch for ten to fifteen seconds. Try it with both knees. Once is enough.

SECOND EXERCISE

BENT-KNEE SIT-UPS

Lie with raised knees; tighten your abdomen, contracting these muscles to their maximum effort; and press your back flat. Cross your arms on your chest, and raise your head and shoulders several inches off the bed if you can. It is these first inches, an angle of not more than thirty degrees, that shorten your abdominals. Do not even aim to arrive at a sitting position despite the name of the

FREE Weight Loss Book!

BUSINESS REPLY MAIL
FIRST CLASS MAIL   PERMIT NO. 79SC   EMMAUS, PA

POSTAGE WILL BE PAID BY ADDRESSEE

PREVENTION®

BOX 202
EMMAUS, PA 18099-0202

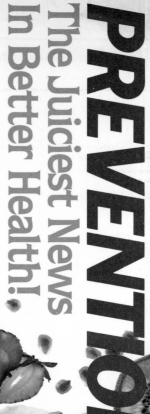

PREVENTION®

The Juiciest News In Better Health!

One Year Subscription—
12 Issues—$15.97 PLUS The
No Diet, No Willpower Way to
Weight Loss Book—FREE!

66526

Name_____

Address_____Apt.#_____

City_____

State_____Zip_____

SEND NO MONEY NOW. JUST MAIL THIS CARD TODAY!

P7333

exercise. Coming to a full sitting position requires the use of muscles other than your abdominals. These muscles, attached to your lower back, can be strained by doing full sit-ups.

Maintain the raised position for a few seconds if you can, and then relax. Try it several times.

To increase the degree of difficulty, leave your arms at your sides. To maximize the challenge to your abdominals, fold your arms behind your head before you do the sit-up. Do not pull your head toward with your arms—this may hurt your neck. Always keep your chin down to permit you to maintain the pelvic tilt.

THIRD EXERCISE

BENT-KNEE SIT-UPS WITH KNEES APART

Many people prefer this exercise to the preceding sit-up with knees together.

Allow your raised knees to fall to the side, tighten your abdomen as you press your back against the bed, and let your chin drop before raising your head and shoulders. Raise only your head and shoulders, and come up not more than thirty degrees. Hold for three or four seconds and drop back.

Do the same exercise with your knees apart and the soles of your feet together. This stretches your adductor, or inner thigh muscles.

Now, with knees apart and abdomen tight, contract your buttocks as tightly as you can and do the sit-up. Repeat several times, more as you become able. THIS MAY BE THE ONE MOST EFFECTIVE EXERCISE YOU EVER DO. IF YOU DO ONLY ONE EXERCISE, LET YOUR KNEES ROLL APART, TIGHTEN YOUR ABDOMEN, TIGHTEN YOUR BUTTOCKS, AND RAISE YOUR

HEAD AND SHOULDERS! If tightening your buttocks causes back pain, you will have to wait before starting this. Then make it a priority. This one exercise combines the benefits of several. Do it daily for the rest of your life, whether you do it for ten repetitions or do it only once.

FOURTH EXERCISE
KEGEL OR PELVIC FLOOR EXERCISE

This is usually included only in childbirth classes, where its importance is more obvious. However, the Kegel exercise emphasizes the importance of including tight buttocks when doing the sit-up. The Kegel, named for its physician discoverer more than forty-five years ago, tightens the circular sphincter muscles around body openings and the supporting tissues of the pelvic floor in both men and women.

Often when people tighten the buttocks they automatically tighten the muscle tissues of the pelvic floor, the area between the thighs composed of both muscle and connective tissue. Upon the pelvic floor rests the weight of the internal organs while one is in the standing or sitting positions. The pelvic floor can sag, or it can be drawn up to control body openings. A stream of urine can be interrupted by controlling these muscles. Backache may be only indirectly related to a weak pelvic floor and the resulting effect on internal organs and their ligaments, but strengthening it is one more way of protecting your back. This exercise has been used to treat urinary incontinence, to aid in childbirth, to treat female sexual dysfunction, and now to treat back ailments.

Draw up the pelvic floor as if to prevent emptying the rectum or bladder over a count of six, and release over a count of six. It can be done with or without tight buttocks. To make sure you differentiate between the two muscle groups—pelvic floor and buttocks—you can do the exercise both ways. With no one the wiser, you can do it anytime, anyplace. If you are pregnant, this exercise is essential, and you should do it at least several times each day to strengthen and gain control over the muscles of your vagina.

FIFTH EXERCISE
CURL-UPS

These are easily confused with sit-ups and with knee-to-chest stretches. In a sense they are a combination of both.

Again, on your back, draw up your knees and tighten your abdomen, with your feet resting on the bed. This time raise your head and shoulders, and, at the same time, with your arms wrapped around your knees, draw your knees toward your nose. Do this, as always, slowly and smoothly. Hold for a few seconds and release.

For more stretch, place your hands under your knees instead of around them. Later you can do one knee at a time, bringing it toward the opposite shoulder for a diagonal action. There are no hard facts on when to start this. Timing depends on your back and your fitness level as well as your preference. Among Level Three exercises, additional diagonal exercises will be offered.

SIXTH EXERCISE
WALL SLIDES

Yes, wall slides. The purpose of this exercise is to strengthen your quadriceps muscles, the front ones in your thighs. You need strong quads to assist you in standing and walking. They are essential if you are to rise correctly from a chair, if you plan to bend or lift anything at all. Without strong quads it is all too easy to bend and lift using your lower back muscles to favor the upper thighs.

You started your exercise program by strengthening abdominals and stretching your back and hamstrings

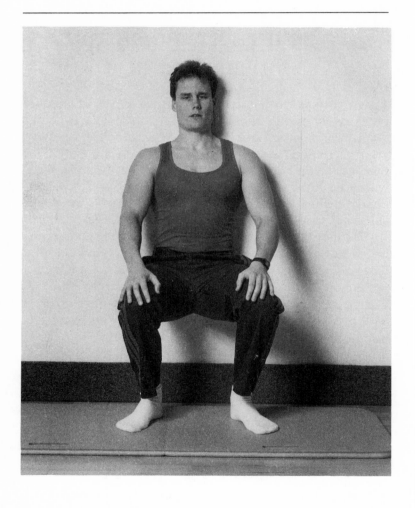

□ Level Two. Wall Slide

without gravitational pull. This upright exercise places less strain on your back than does standing because you are leaning against a wall. It does require that you have learned the pelvic tilt and stretched your hamstrings.

Back up to a wall with your feet approximately two feet from it, the distance about that of the length of your thighs. Your arms should be at your sides. Flatten your back against the wall as you assume the pelvic tilt and slowly slide down the wall, maintaining your back flat against it until your thighs are parallel to the floor. Hold the position a few seconds if you can, longer if possible. If you cannot hold it more than a second or two, do several repetitions instead.

SEVENTH EXERCISE

LEG RAISES, VARIATIONS ON THE THEME

Many back exercise sheets include single or even double straight-leg raising, while others suggest that you do no leg-raising at all in the supine, lying-on-your-back position, the usual position for leg-raising.

The risks are described as straining your lower back muscles. The benefits described by others are stretching hamstrings, tightening abdominals, and strengthening your thighs. To sort out the apparent discrepancies, the lower back is strained if the abdominal muscles cannot hold the pelvic tilt with legs straight and raised. Raising both legs is still more difficult to do but easier to remember. However, there appear to be better ways to strengthen abdominals and stretch hamstrings as well as to strengthen the thighs.

Other exercise sheets—the majority—suggest bending the knees, then straightening them as you raise them to the vertical position, then bending them again as you lower them, doing this one leg at a time. Or they suggest raising your legs perpendicular to the bed and lowering them until you begin to lose the pelvic tilt. The benefit to your back comes from the first few degrees of lowering. Once you lose the tilt you begin to hurt your back.

This is the way it works: As you lower your straightened legs from the vertical position toward the horizontal, the first third of the descent uses your abdominal muscles. As you continue to lower your legs, the active muscles are those attached from the front of your thighs to your lower back. These are not particularly strong, and there can be considerable pull on your lower back, and consequent injury. And during those first thirty degrees of descent, as stated, your abdominals must be strong enough to hold your back flat. The angle is everything, or almost everything.

Many in back exercise classes report that they forgot how to do the leg raises and were not sure they were doing them right. Even more important, if they do not like the exercise and view it as a chore, it and other exercises may be ignored. Lack of compliance with even some of the few exercises generally offered to patients has proved a major obstacle for back sufferers and health care personnel treating them and can only contribute to chronic problems.

Here are two variations that are pleasant, simple, and effective:

1. Stand with your side to the wall and your hand supporting your balance on the wall. Tighten your abdomen as you assume the pelvic tilt. Swing forward your straightened leg, the leg away from the wall, pointing with your heel, not your toe. The leg is raised only as high as is comfortable for you. The position is not maintained, but held only momentarily, and the swing is repeated. This exercise with pointed heel helps to stretch tight calf muscles. Done with pointed toe, you can get a muscle cramp in your calf.

The same exercise is performed by placing your opposite hand on the wall and again swinging forward the outside leg.

In the upright position the gravitational pull on your lower back is less than in the supine when you are doing leg raising. This is an exercise you

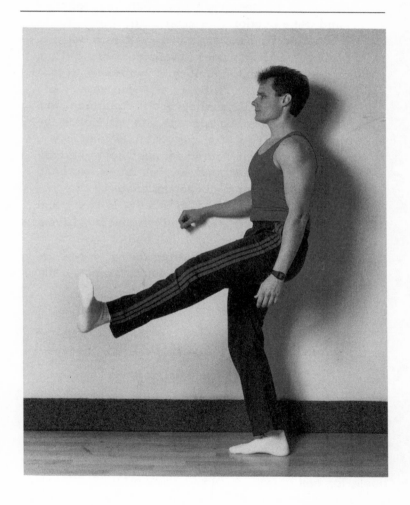

Level Two. Standing Leg Raise

can do almost anywhere, anyplace, including your office. You may find this exercise useful, especially if you are at work and feel the beginnings of back spasm.

2. This exercise is similar to the standard ones but easier to remember, pleasanter to do, and has some added benefits. You do both legs together and get a comfortable inner thigh stretch, too.

Lie on your flattened back with raised knees. Bring your bent knees toward your chest. Then straighten them, pointing with your heels, to your point of tension. Probably your hamstrings and calf muscles will not allow you to straighten them entirely, but as you practice you will notice the increased stretch. You get benefit as long as you feel some stretch. Your knees need not be straight unless this occurs because your calves and hamstrings have already been stretched.

Now stretch them apart in a "v" to your point of comfort. Bring them together, and bend them before replacing them on the bed.

Later you can try lowering the "v" a few degrees as long as you can maintain the pelvic tilt. Do what is comfortable for you.

EIGHTH EXERCISE
EASY CALF STRETCH

Stand with your toes on a step, lowering your heels until you feel tension in your lower leg muscles as you balance yourself with a railing. Especially if you are a female accustomed to wearing shoes with high or moderately high heels, the calf muscles may be short and tight, contributing to back pain. In any case, these muscles need to be stretched regularly. Tight calf muscles are impediments to bending and lifting, leading to the inappropriate use of lower back muscles for these tasks.

The easy way to do this is simply to stand with your feet flat on the floor and bend your knees to the point of

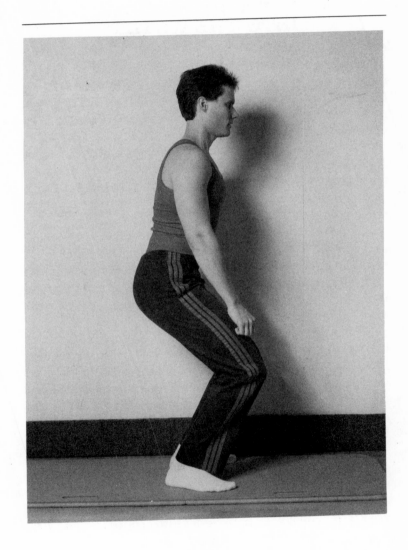

Level Two. Easy Calf Stretch

tension in your calf muscles. You can do this almost any-time and anyplace. You do not need to have stairs.

OUT OF THE HOUSE AND INTO THE WATER

You may have heard that swimming is good for your back because you are weightless in the water. You do not know just why that is important exactly, nor what kind of swimming stroke is recommended or how to use the water most effectively.

How soon, or if, you use a pool or lake for your back recovery program depends on your preference, and also the difficulty and possible inconvenience of getting there. However, swimming can be a great stress reliever if you can manage it.

In the water you can try out motions you might hesitate to try on land because you are not dealing with gravity, and also because you cannot make fast motions you might later regret. Water offers resistance to your muscular activity and therefore can offer aerobic benefit as you walk and eventually even jog in the water.

Diving, however, carries its own risks, including arching your back. The Australian crawl swimming stroke also involves arching your back, a position you should avoid until you feel able, and that can be weeks or months. Even if you are weightless, do not twist in the water until you are ready, which will be after you can begin to extend your back into a modified arch.

Take care not to slip on the wet edges of the pool as you enter. Start by floating on your back, and sculling with your arms, or even wearing a flotation device, such as a water ski belt, if you wish, so you do not have to kick your legs at all if your back is still sore. Your arms and legs are bent in a froglike position.

When you are certain you can keep your buttocks

tucked under in the pelvic tilt, you can stretch out to float on your back with buttocks tucked under and your abdomen tight. Tighten your buttocks, and hold for several seconds. Stretch your arms above your head as you continue to float. If you need to move your legs to remain afloat, bend your knees slightly before you kick. Finally, float with tilted pelvis, your arms straight above your head, and kick gently with straight knees. This last activity may not be possible for some time.

Start kicking with bent knees, whatever you may have learned in early swimming classes. Only later can you straighten them when you have stronger hip, thigh, and abdominal muscles. Sculling on your back can give you some arm and shoulder strength, and moving your legs, even with no significant water resistance, gives circulatory benefit. At first the less kicking you do the better, because kicking can irritate the tissues in your back.

From this you can move to the elementary backstroke and then the backstroke. The crawl comes later, especially the crawl combined with the kicking motion, and finally the breaststroke.

When you leave the pool, grasp the handrails, and with your body still in the water, walk up the steps to place yourself in a knee-to-chest or fetal position. Relax in this position a few seconds for a gentle stretch before climbing out of the pool.

Swimming can be a welcome change, especially when just about every recreational sport you can think of is all but impossible.

CHAPTER SEVEN
UP-AND-ABOUT
BACK PROTECTION

□

Whether you have had a scary bout with acute back pain or have had periodic mild backaches, you should now be confident that you can prevent the possibility of becoming suddenly disabled for an indefinite period of time.

The "core exercises" are those presented in Level One and Level Two. Chapter Eight will give you the Level Three exercises to provide the final step. You have not yet worked directly on strengthening your back and other important muscles. Nor have you yet done the stretches that can enormously improve your sense of well-being, besides offering you still more back protection. In the meantime, you need to know how to go about your daily life without harming your back.

You are back at the office, back at school, back making business trips. The ways in which you move are critical. Remember that you can make an occasional mistake, and the stronger your back, the less disastrous a false move is likely to be, even though habitual postural errors increase risk of back pain recurrence. This information may help you to hold your back less rigidly, permitting the muscles to relax.

In practice, the fact that you do the back exercises helps to ensure that you remember to move in ways that will strengthen and protect your back. Some common incorrect motions are associated with the weak, tight muscles of an inadequate back strengthening program.

STANDING TIPS

While you stand, your back is best protected while neither arched nor flexed, but maintained in a normal shallow curve. Only in this position with the pelvis under the spine do the broad pelvic bones support the spinal column with maximum effectiveness.

The well-shod foot for a back pain sufferer means flat shoes rather than raised heels. Raised heels throw your body out of alignment and increase the arch in your lower back. Boots that come up over your ankles are a hindrance rather than a help to a sore back. Crepe soles instead of leather soles on your shoes cushion pavement shock and add welcome comfort as you walk. Sneakers do the same.

Socks or bare feet permit desirable toe action and contact with the floor unless you have a slippery floor surface. Sandals and slingback shoes will make your contact with the floor less sure, increasing muscle tension in your back.

Standing can be tiring even with a strong back. Remaining in one position encourages muscle fatigue and back muscle spasm in particular; when fatigued abdominals relax, you lose your pelvic tilt. Move around as much as you can. In elevators stand with your feet several inches from the wall, and lean against it, flattening your back as you do so. The wall of a room, a pillar, or a post serves to relieve backache. When you have to stand you can place one foot on a step or stair to prevent back arching and relieve pain.

At first, use elevators instead of stairs. Going upstairs or downstairs often irritates the structures of your back. Instead, replace that activity with back exercises.

RULES TO BEND BY: "KNEES UNDER YOUR NOSE"

"Bend and touch your fingers to the floor." At one time toe-touching was a staple exercise. It is still found in exercise books and in exercise classes. It appears as a simple back stretch, warm-up, and "get the blood to the head." If you are young and your upper body is not heavy and your back is strong, you may have no apparent problem, but you still put your back at risk, if not now, then in the future, by continuing to bend with straight knees. In effect, you are folding yourself in half at the waist, one of the worst things you can do, especially in the standing position. Do not touch your toes.

Do not bend forward at all from your waist. Do not bend over the drinking fountain, the crib, or the sink to brush your teeth, nor to enter your car, whatever the current state of your back. There is another way.

You have heard of people who bent forward to bow from the waist and "threw their backs out." Occasionally they could not even straighten up after bowing. This occurrence appeared so bizarre and incomprehensible that it could only contribute to the perception that there is just no rhyme or reason to back pain. In fact, bowing hurts your back. Curtsying does not! Why?

Bending from the waist requires that your back muscles have enough power to hoist erect the weight of your upper body. As they contract in the attempt to lift this substantial load, they can go into spasm. It is not so much the forward motion by itself as it is the attempt to straighten that strains your back. But maintaining even a slight forward bend is hard on your back. If you twist your body as you straighten, you place more strain on your back. And if, as you straighten, you are also lifting a carton of soup cans, the strain is further intensified. If the carton, as it is lifted, is held away from your body instead of close to your body, and your back is arched when you straighten, the intensity of the strain on your back is greatest of all. You strain muscles and ligaments. The extraordinary pressures on the discs if you use your back as a lever may result in a herniated or ruptured disc. This "lift with a twist" may seem at first, until you think about it, rather unimportant.

If you find yourself bent forward before you straighten, brace your hands on your knees and walk them up your thighs as you draw yourself erect. Better yet, bend your knees before you attempt to straighten.

Bending correctly is good for your back. You have already done bending in the supine, on-your-back position and on your side. Later, doing it on your feet can be beneficial, too, because it does stretch your lower back, rotates your hip joints, and also strengthens your thigh and abdominal muscles when performed in a way to protect your back. Having done the wall slide exercise in Level Two, your legs are prepared to help you bend and later to lift.

When you bend either forward or backward you place substantial pressure on the discs. Although you will not plan to do backbends, it is easy to arch your back inadvertently. During the day you will quite constantly bend forward, but, as long as you bring your knees ahead of your back as you bend, your back is protected.

"Bend your knees" has long been the exhortation when explaining proper procedure for bending and lifting. Instead, think "knees in front of back" to remind yourself of the reason. When you stand, your knees are under your hips. As you bend, your knees are brought in front of your hips and shoulders to protect your back. As you bend, your knees are higher than your hips. Say to yourself, "knees under nose, knees ahead of nose, or knees ahead of hips."

How does bending work in practice? You drop down into a squatting or fetal position, or drop into a kneeling position. The former requires adequate calf muscle stretch; the latter requires adequate stretch in the front muscles of your thighs. Your task may not require that you bend all the way down to the floor. In this case you flex your knees as needed, and use your hand to brace yourself, perhaps on a piece of furniture if your shoulders start to come ahead of your knees. Getting back up requires strength in your front thigh muscles known as quadriceps.

As you bend, your back is straight but not arched. It can angle forward as long as your knees remain in front of your hips and shoulders. Do not twist your knees to the side. Do not drop your shoulders to produce an excessive "C-shaped" curve. If you do, you may put excessive stress on ligaments and tendons as well as on discs.

Both custom and wearing tight clothes have contributed to the habit of pitching the shoulders forward, ignoring the hip joints, and keeping knees straight and close together. Many people do not have the muscle stretch required to drop down as they bend, nor enough strength in their legs to get back up. These two factors combine to encourage folding themselves in half as they bend from the waist instead of using knee and hip joints designed for bending. And the quadriceps muscles become weaker and tighter rather than stronger and more flexible.

CRIBS AND DRINKING FOUNTAINS: WHAT ABOUT THE FURNITURE?

1. To spread a blanket or sheet on your bed, either sit on the bed or kneel. Or bend your knees, brac-

ing them against the edge of the bed for support. Many ruptured discs have occurred with bed-making as the apparent precipitating factor. Kneeling on the floor and sitting back on your heels with straight back is the preferred position and very safe for your back.

2. Approaching a drinking fountain requires ingenuity. You can do a modified forward lunge, keeping one knee ahead of your back. You can place one foot on a stool to help protect your back. You can bend your knees slightly, bracing them against the water cooler. You can place one hand or forearm on the cooler to put some of the force on your arm instead of your back, bending your knees at least slightly, and preferably bracing them against the cooler.

   An alternative is to collect the water into a paper cup.

3. Infant cribs win the prize for the worst-designed item of furniture for caregivers' backs, even strong backs. Supermarket carriages are a close second. Women who have recently given birth have had their abdominal muscles stretched, and their ligaments and joints weakened by the hormones of pregnancy. Not only does the crib encourage parents to bend with straight knees, but also they must then lift the baby, and the lift is not the recommended close-to-the-body lift as they reach over the edge of the crib. The scene is set for strain, sprain, and disc damage.

   Draw in the abdominals and place one leg up on a footstool, an upended wastebasket, or a couple of thick telephone books. Lean your forearms on the edge of the crib. Drop the crib sides before lifting the baby.

   Women who have had back injuries as a result of their use of cribs or low changing tables, or hunching over a sink have not infrequently spent weeks and longer lying on mats on the floor with their babies, or on their beds with babies, unable to use the crib at all. Change your baby by placing him or her on a blanket on the floor and kneeling for the diaper changes.

4. Brush your teeth by bringing the toothbrush up to your mouth instead of bending, or use a footstool and rest a forearm on the edge of the sink.

5. Tie your shoes by sitting in a chair for balance and bending forward to reach over your flexed knees. Your shoulders are over your knees, not ahead of them.

6. You can do a bend with your shoulders coming somewhat forward of your knees by bracing your back with both hands on your knees.

7. Lifting anything out of your car trunk or the car interior can be difficult. Kneeling is best, but more practical is putting one knee ahead of your nose.

8. Get into the car either by placing your hands first on the seat, or put one knee ahead of your back. Easiest is turning away from the car, sitting on the seat, and then swinging your legs into the car.

LIFTING LOGIC: LESS IS BEST

Lifting in general is not beneficial to your back. Later—much later, after a back attack—lifting objects may serve to strengthen instead of injuring muscles, ligaments, and discs, but this could be a year or longer, or never, depending on your situation. For some people lifting is never a health-promoting activity, if, for example, there is serious disc damage. Back muscles can be strengthened in Level Three without, in the process, involving the vertical compressive force of gravity on the discs.

Lifting requires back muscles, abdominal muscles, leg muscles, and shoulder, arm, and neck muscles. All can be strengthened without carrying packages, children, or furniture.

If you are recovering from a back pain episode, the advice is, from all sources, to lift absolutely nothing. This recommendation appears sound because back sufferers who do lift report rapid onset of pain and fatigue, as might be expected from the anatomy and mechanics involved. When you can start to lift and carry depends on your back, the strength of the abdominals in particular, but other muscles as well, and the time required to reabsorb ruptured disc material, or heal muscles and ligaments. You may have injury to all three tissues. Talk with your doctor.

Typically, progress in ability to lift covers a long time span, even if you have moved quickly in your proficiency with Level One and Level Two exercises. These two levels and the body mechanics so far presented cannot hurt your back unless you have a disabling medical condition, or accident, or try to stretch tight back muscles too fast. At first there may have been so much back irritation that you could barely move at all and remained lying on your side. Bending need not stress your back. Lifting does.

Your back muscles have contracted and been strengthened as you stand and walk. The Level One and Level Two exercises such as curl-ups and sit-ups do not strengthen back muscles. Fatigue or the onset of discomfort have been your guide as you stood and walked. In most situations of back pain there is no other.

When starting, try to lift less than you can. Stop at the first sign of fatigue or strain. Problems may not be evident for several hours if you have pushed the limit, so it is preferable to stop well before you feel any discomfort at all.

1. Start with only a couple of pounds. Always assume the pelvic tilt before you lift. Hold the weight close to the midpoint of your body at waist level.

2. Divide the load if you can into two parcels of equal weight. For example, it is better to carry a half gallon of milk with your left arm and a half gallon using your right arm than to carry a single gallon jug.

3. Some loads are better carried on your back, such as a child or your luggage.

4. Push or pull an object instead of lifting wherever possible.

5. With your feet pointing directly toward it, face the object you will lift. Turn your feet, not your upper body, so that you will never twist as you lift. Your legs and abdominal muscles are used in lifting.

6. Try not to lift an object above your waist. If you must put something on a high shelf, first put one foot on a stool to prevent your back from arching. You are trying to avoid arching your back, and certainly lifting is the worst time to do so.

7. Learn to bend before you lift. Follow the Rules to Bend by. Of course, do not bend from the waist to lift. If you did, you would be adding the weight of your upper body to the object you are lifting!

8. Squat, or better still, kneel before lifting. An alternative is to place one foot forward and lower yourself slowly to the other knee. The front foot, which should be flat on the floor, will be used for lifting. The rear foot, flexed at the toes, will serve for pushing and balance.

9. Raising window sashes has been disastrous for countless back sufferers. Impatience compounds the problem. If you must do it, follow all the rules and have sticky windows fixed.

SITTING AND LIKING IT

After learning that sitting places one and half times more stress on your back than standing or walking, you should not feel dismayed that it takes so long before you can sit for a reasonable length of time. Like lifting, avoid it for as long as necessary, because sitting does nothing to strengthen or increase back fitness in any way. Sitting can hurt your back and delay your recovery. It can be especially difficult if you have had a herniated or ruptured disc.

A common misconception is that the next step after bed rest is sitting up. When that causes pain, the patients go home from their offices and back to bed! And they do not even think of doing the prescribed exercises!

Driving a car can be even more discouraging because it places more stress on your back than simply sitting. Riding as a passenger in a car or bus can cause severe pain unless you can lie down or have a seat that reclines.

Use the following coping strategies. Especially, choose your chair.

1. Pick a chair with armrests, and use the armrests. This helps to remove some of the weight from your lower spine as the weight of your arms is eliminated. You can use the chair arms to lift yourself up, shifting your weight at intervals.

2. Avoid sitting on a soft bed or soft chairs. The unstable, unsupportive surface tends to cause back muscles to contract and go into spasm.

3. Rocking chairs can relieve back pain by changing the angle of inclination so that your muscles are not held in one position. As you rock you can remove a portion of gravitational forces, especially as you rock backward.

4. The chair must have a back, and there should not be an open space at the lumbar region. Your lower back should be supported to hold it at the correct angle, not swayed or overly rounded, and the seat should be firm. You should be able to vary the angle of inclination. The chair can be molded plastic or upholstered. The wedge pillow you use in your car can be a big help in the office, too. Place the large part of the wedge at the base of the backrest. A folded towel can be used.

5. Your feet should be able to rest flat on the floor. If not, your back will tend to arch. If the front part of the seat is slightly higher than the back part of the seat, the comfort for many people is increased. If your knees are raised higher than your hips, you may improve your comfort level. Place your feet on a horizontal wastebasket or several telephone books. Placing even one foot on a stool will help. The chair should be deep enough to support the entire thigh. Rest your forearms on your chair or on your desk.

6. Get up and walk frequently.

7. Balance chairs, with some of your weight resting on your knees, are comfortable for many unless they have problem knees. They have no backs, but the alignment of your spine is correct. You can try one out in a store and ascertain its comfort relatively quickly. Many like them so much they bring them to work.

8. With few exceptions, seats in cars and planes are notoriously poorly designed for back comfort, even when they can be reclined. In most, both the seat and the lower backrest have inadequate support. Place a pillow at your lower back in a plane or in the car. Buy a wedge-shaped plastic pillow. It is easy to carry with you and is designed to support your back. Wedges are available in auto

supply stores and are carried by many chain stores. The thick portion of the wedge is placed at the bottom, with the thinner part above.

9. Do not slump in your chair unless you wedge a pillow firmly in the space this creates between the chair and your back. Slumping can place strain on discs and ligaments. A better plan is to recline your chair. When you get into your car, tilt your pelvis before you settle against your cushion and the seat of the car. From time to time as you sit, raise your shoulders, tighten your abdominals and buttocks for several seconds, and then release.

10. When you drive, bring your car seat forward so that your leg is extended as little as possible while you drive. An extended leg strains your back because you tend to lose the pelvic tilt, and can increase sciatic pain as well. You can recline your seat backward as far as you feel is safe. However, make sure that your vision of the road ahead and behind is unimpaired. A reclining angle of up to 120 degrees increases back comfort.

11. There is a difference of opinion on whether to cross your knees as you sit. Most practitioners tend to discourage it because it places uneven stress on muscles and may strain ligaments. Others say it helps to guarantee that the pelvic tilt will be maintained.

12. Get up from your chair by pushing on the chair armrests and using your upper thigh muscles.

SAVING YOUR NECK

When you think of it as you sit or stand or walk, tuck in your chin and stretch out the back of your neck, then return your chin to a position parallel to the floor. Your neck may tend to get sore if you let your head settle into your shoulders like a turtle for prolonged periods, or if you let it hang forward for long stretches of time.

If you lie in bed with your head pushed forward, you invite damage to neck structures, so instead arrange pillows in a layered, shingled design to help keep your head aligned with your raised shoulders. Sometimes neck collars are used to help remind people to pay attention to the position in which they hold their necks.

TRAVEL TIPS

1. Use soft-sided luggage, including garment bags.

2. To avoid carrying a larger bag, divide the load into two smaller bags.

3. Use luggage with wheels. Use shoulder bags.

4. Caring for your back is just one more reason to travel light.

5. Get up, change position often. Do not remain sitting for long periods.

6. Avoid lifting anything with any weight into overhead luggage racks.

7. Allow adequate time for everything.

8. Wear comfortable shoes and clothing.

9. Continue an exercise program.

10. Plan for time to relax.

CHAPTER EIGHT
LEVEL THREE: THE ICING ON THE CAKE

☐

Level Three is, in fact, far more than "the icing on the cake." What you discover here represents the path toward total back fitness.

A fit back helps you to sit without discomfort on a backless stool at a lunch counter and to stand in line at a movie theater. Can you sit on a backless stadium bench for more than a short while? Without bracing your elbows on your knees? Back strength helps avoid fatigue and consequent back muscle spasm. A fit back, both strong and flexible, can more easily withstand the stress of a fall or injury, or the injuries resulting from repetitive motions. It helps sports performance whether in hiking, basketball, or tennis. Back fitness should be taught beginning in elementary schools, both the techniques and the "whys."

KNOWING THE TERMS

Learn the meaning of the words. Some terms are old, some are new.

1. *Supine* means lying on your back.

2. *Prone* means lying on your abdomen.

3. *Stretch* means lengthening of muscles.

4. *Contract* means shortening muscle length, as occurs when a muscle is worked.

5. *Flex* means to bend a joint. *Flexing* your back means bending it forward. When bending forward, your knees are also *flexed,* meaning bent, to protect your back. *Flexion* exercises bring your back forward in the direction of your knees.

6. *Pelvic tilt* means flattened curve of the lower back, abdominal muscles contracted, and buttocks tucked down and under the spine.

7. *Extend* means to straighten a joint. *Back extension* exercises are the opposite of the *pelvic tilt.* The back is straightened and *arched.* The *arched* back occurring in *back extension* exercises enhances temporarily the natural curve of the lower back.

8. *Hyperextension* is described as an overly arched back, as in gymnastics and backbends.

"ARCH THAT BACK"

Now is time to learn to arch your back—yes, arch your back, the very opposite of the pelvic tilt learned in Levels One and Two on the preceding pages. This, after all you have learned about the pelvic tilt and the need to reduce the curve in your lower back, to flatten your back always as much as possible, both during exercises and in your daily life as you sit, drive, stand, and walk. You probably feel bewildered. You may even be reminded of the apparent contradiction when those with back pain are admonished in the same breath both to rest and to exercise. The rule in Level Three is "keep the pelvic tilt," but also, sometimes, "arch that back."

But wait. Do not arch your back yet. And do not anticipate any suggestion to return to the swaybacked posture, ever.

Once the important pelvic tilt has been learned and practiced, back comfort usually is increased markedly. The result appears almost magical when you stand during a party or museum tour with a tired, actually sore, back. Then, by tightening abdomen and buttocks, perhaps assisted by placing one foot on a stair, the increased pelvic tilt relieves much of your pain in seconds. All this helps to protect the back but not to strengthen it.

It is a real achievement to have learned in Levels One and Two to stretch back muscles, hamstrings, and inner thigh and calf muscles and to strengthen thigh, buttock, and pelvic floor muscles besides tightening those ever-weak abdominal muscles. All of this progress helps make possible your increased comfort and confidence that your back will not let you down.

Sometimes the pelvic tilt, once learned, becomes so pronounced that the pelvis is thrust forward, with shoulders forward and down. The chest tends to cave inward, and the lower back has an outward curve as in the previously described "amateur ice skater's stance." In this position, although the back does not tend to hurt, as it might if it were hollowed and swayed, it appears stiff and inflexible, as described in Chapter Six. If the outward curve is exaggerated into a "C" configuration, the ligaments supporting spinal bones can be overstretched and a force is produced, similar to squeezing a tube of toothpaste, that tends to extrude the disc backward.

Sitting hunched over on a backless stool, instead of keeping the back straight while sitting, brings into play these same undesirable forces on discs and back ligaments.

An overly arched back or a back maintained in an

arched position results in stress on both discs and facet joints. When the spine is bent back upon itself in a pronounced arch, a condition may result that has been described as "kissing spines."

However, the constantly maintained pelvic tilt, even if the rib cage is raised in the correct alignment, results in a flattened, rigid back described in Chapter Six, the appearance more one of aging than that of a strong, fit back.

The person with a history of back pain may say that this unchanging position offers the most security. There is fear of hurting the back by attempting to introduce flexibility. Flexibility is not usually even seen as a goal. For the person with a "bad back" there is often real and understandable fear, as described in Chapter Six, of introducing even the possibility of arch. The vision appears of the arched back with "bone grinding against bone," tightened back muscles, flaccid abdominals, and painful pressure on nerves. An arched back is associated with muscle spasm, which back care programs are designed to relieve.

Only within the past several years has modified arching been introduced at all in any back program. Prior to this time the Williams flexion exercises (named for Paul Williams, who developed them in the 1960s) were the only ones offered. These include the forward-bending curl-ups, modified sit-ups, and knee-chest positions included in Levels One and Two.

Shortly before 1980 Robin McKenzie, an English physician, began recommending moderate back arching. This sparked a debate in print between two well-known physical therapists in the field of pregnancy and postpartum exercise. Back programs have only begun to introduce "bridging" in which, while lying on your back, the knees are raised and the buttocks lifted off the floor.

During pregnancy, bridging probably should be the only back extension exercise you practice. Pregnancy is not the time to initiate back arching when the heavy abdomen is already tending to pull the spine into a swayback position that frequently causes back muscle spasm and increased disc pressures. Someone who is not pregnant but who is overweight with a large abdomen might do well to concentrate instead on the pelvic tilt and to minimize back arching.

Bridging sometimes is listed as a buttock-firming exercise, but there are better ones for this. Athletic trainers, while stressing the importance of flexion exercises, are including bridging and sometimes another extension exercise as well.

The Williams and McKenzie approaches appear to be directly contradictory, and in a sense they are. The Williams approach encourages elimination of the curve in the lower back to the maximum possible extent. The McKenzie approach stresses the importance of maintaining a moderate lower back curve, describing this more in terms of maintaining an improved balance of pressures on the discs than in terms of a strong back, although this is what results, as back muscles are contracted to form the arch.

The literature describes a study of these two apparently divergent approaches. One group of back pain sufferers was given exercises based on the Williams principles, and the other was given back extension exercises representing the McKenzie approach. The results favored the latter. It was a preliminary study and, as will be described in Chapter Nine, studies on back pain have a number of inherent difficulties.

The bottom line seems to be that you need both types of exercises, first the so-called flexion, or Williams, exercises and later, to a somewhat lesser extent, you need to include back extension exercises. In the absence of a major medical problem, you will decide how much of each and when. Excessive back extension almost inevitably will cause you to bring your knees to your chest into a position of flexion. A strong, flexible back seems to require both types of exercises. As you continue to understand better your body and your back, the two approaches become less contradictory than they may at first appear.

The range of useful back extension exercises will be described in two sections of this chapter, the one on stretching and the section on developing back strength. When you are ready to do back extension, these arching exercises and body positions can feel very good to your back, not something you "ought" to do.

Occasionally, without your conscious plan, you wake up one morning after dutifully sleeping on your side for weeks to find yourself on your stomach. Or you are in the pool doing your backstroke, while carefully maintaining your pelvic tilt, and you find yourself wanting to flip over and do the crawl. You have not made an error. Your back may be giving you a sign that it is ready for Level Three.

WHAT? NO BACK EXERCISES YET?

So far you have not done any back exercises. Not that you have not used your back muscles at all. They are involved in walking and in keeping you upright while you stand. But sit-ups, curl-ups, wall slides, pelvic rocks on all fours, and all the others in Level One and Level Two can be practiced for months without making your back one bit stronger. Many people think they have gone through a back care program, but actually they have not done a single back exercise.

Whether this has occurred by design or by default, it is not possible to exercise a sore back, whether the problem is strain, sprain, or a disc problem, all of which may result in back muscle spasm. Irritation, pain, and possible small muscle and ligament tears may require weeks or possibly months after a back attack before actual back strengthening exercises can be initiated, even though Levels One and Two exercises can and should begin earlier. Persistent practice of Levels One and Two exercises tend to shorten the time required before you are ready for back exercises. Depending on your medical diagnosis and history, you may want to consult your medical provider before starting them. Level Three assumes a basically healthy back.

A muscle cannot be required to work if it has not first been stretched. That you began when you stretched your back in Level One.

And to work a muscle means to contract it. To contract it means shortening its length. When your back muscles are contracted, your tilted pelvis changes its alignment into an arched configuration. Back exercises therefore result in arching your back. Back exercises are "extension" exercises, whereas up to now you have been focusing on "flexion" exercises.

THEN WHY GO ON TO INCLUDE BACK EXERCISES AT ALL?

Your well back *needs* to be arched sometimes, that is why! Your back muscles require conditioning. Most of the time your back maintains the pelvic tilt to avoid stressing your lower back discs and back joints, but not always.

The preceding exercises have served to improve the postural alignment so vital in protecting your back from the effects of a predominantly sedentary life-style and in avoiding injury during daily activities and sports.

Your strong abdomen helps to brace your back. Stronger buttock and thigh muscles help to support your back and ensure that you can bend and lift safely. The exaggerated lower back arch, straining all the structures of the lower back, has been modified. Your pelvis is now located under your spine, not in back of it, to stabilize your back better. Your discs are better protected now that your back is aligned in its natural shallow curves.

You have learned to relax tight muscles. Your back is

stretched, and its supporting muscles in the legs and buttocks have been strengthened. If you had pain when you started your back program, it is now gone. But do not stop here, even though you feel you are managing just fine. Besides avoiding back fatigue, there are other reasons for working toward achieving a fit back.

Recent findings from the Mayo Clinic reported in a monthly digest of medical facts and news (see the Bibliography), indicate a positive correlation between back strength and decreased spinal osteoporosis. "The density and amount of calcium in an older woman's spinal bones correlates very closely with the strength of her back muscles." (*Mayo Clinic Proceedings* 61:116 [1986]). This is just one more reason for strengthening your back.

The need for a graduated exercise program has been stated in a business journal article, by two pain centers for those with back problems (see the Bibliography). At the University of Miami Comprehensive Pain and Rehabilitation Center, 86 percent of seven thousand patients who came to the center for back surgery did not need surgery after a four-week intensive exercise program. The original purpose had been to teach exercises to be performed after the surgery.

Back muscles most likely to be injured are known as the erector spinae, running parallel to the spine on either side of it, from the sacrum to the skull. They consist of three groups of muscles. By strengthening them you increase your protection against back injury. Industry's desire to assess the likelihood of back injury for workers, especially laborers who do repeated lifting, has led to the development of equipment that can measure back muscle fiber activity and strength. The results are expected to be used as a predictor of possible back injury.

Your back has been protected partly by the stretching exercises and also by the forward-bending flexion exercises. In these, your lower back has been straight or slightly curved, your knees have been bent, and your shoulders have been brought forward in the direction of your knees. This has been accomplished by contracting, and therefore strengthening, your longitudinal abdominal muscles, which extend from your sternum, or breastbone, to your pubic bone. Many mistakenly assume the abdominal muscles extend only from the navel to this frontal pubic bone. When you lie on your back and bring forward your shoulders off the floor against gravitational force, you can do this only by working your abdominals. (If you pull up more than a few degrees off the floor, however, muscles connecting your leg and lower back are brought into play, and you may injure your back because of undue work demanded of this muscle group. The back may be pulled into an arch.) The final step after stretching back muscles and strengthening those that protect the back is to condition the back muscles themselves.

"SO WHERE IS YOUR BACKBONE?"

Physically, a strong back results in less fatigue, in confidence in your back so you can allow it safely to be flexible. Remember, flexibility is defined as range of motion of a joint. You can do sidebends and even rotate your back on its axis because the differing anatomy of the thoracic vertebrae in the chest area allows this action. A fit back provides the foundation for any sports program, whether playing tennis, basketball, paddling a canoe, or swinging a baseball bat.

LEVEL THREE IN THREE PARTS

Beginning Level Three exercises means that you have a problem-free back under ordinary circumstances. Your level of aspiration includes more than simply avoiding repeated episodes of back pain.

If you have never had back pain, go through the exercises in the preceding levels to ensure that ongoing abdominal muscle tightening occurs, also buttock tightening, hamstring stretching, and quadriceps strengthening. Do these exercises at least three times per week.

Level Three is comprised of (1) stretching muscles in many parts of your body, especially the postural muscles, followed by (2) back strengthening exercises, and (3) several additional back fitness exercises for enhanced strengthening and flexibility.

Exercises listed in the stretching category cannot help but have also a strengthening component and vice versa. When you shorten one muscle, as previously described, you stretch the opposing muscle group. For example, when you flex (bend) your arm you contract the biceps in the front of your arm. And when you extend (straighten) your arm, especially against some form of resistance such as the arm of your chair, you can feel muscles on the back of your arm, your triceps, tighten. The biceps are now stretched and nonworking (not contracting). Similar principles operate when you flex and extend your leg, your hand, your foot, your body (your back).

Every suggested exercise need not be practiced, even though no one exercise accomplishes exactly what another does. Try each one of the possibilities at least once to become aware of its effects on muscles. Some postures or exercises may be done almost automatically, even several times a day, for comfort. Avoid postures or exercises that cause discomfort or pain. Pick several you like.

Some exercises you simply may not like, while others become favorites. With some guidelines, the choice is yours. Keep in mind that an exercise that appears difficult, or one you do not enjoy, may mean only that the muscles required for the exercise are weak. When they gain strength, your opinion may change.

Increasing the number of repetitions of each is not really the goal, either, and speed is not the goal at all. This is not a calisthenics program in which rapid-fire sit-ups and push-ups are done with a stopwatch. This approach will never help your back and may even do the opposite. Bouncing or jumping activities have a negative effect on your back and other joints. However, just one slow, steady motion, and maintaining the body position for several seconds to your "point of tension" offer a substantial return on this small investment in back fitness.

It is not necessary to set aside unconscionable amounts of time nor to schedule any particular time of day. An inflexible approach can contribute to stress by adding one more "ought to do" to your schedule, an approach that could contribute to discontinuing the program because you cannot take the time.

Your body is not immobile except when you "exercise" it, not even at night during sleep. You move, stretch, and change position. When you awake you continue to move throughout the day.

Not all your motions may be helpful. Sometimes you tense your neck and shoulders for inordinate amounts of time while hunched over your desk.

When seated for prolonged periods of time, bend forward over your knees as if to pick up a paper from the floor to stretch out your back. While sitting in traffic, arch your back momentarily against the seat of the car, giving your back muscles a chance to contract and your chest the opportunity to expand. Take a deep breath and relax your entire body as you exhale. These are only some of the ways to use stretching techniques in daily life.

UNDER ONE ROOF

The need is universal for regular back protection exercises. Readers of this book may range from back pain sufferers who for years have engaged in minimal physical exercise to those who are engaged in high-intensity athletics and want a strong back.

Understanding the issues and the controversies in back care, and, in a later chapter, how medicine comes into the picture put into perspective the range of back exercises.

AN AWESOME ARRAY

The awesome array of exercises, especially in Level Three, is a result of the effort to give a more total picture of the back's requirements for exercise than has been previously available, a chance for total back fitness. Therefore, a wider net has been cast.

In addition, as previously discussed, many disciplines impinge on back health. These include several medical specialities, physical therapy, exercise physiology, sports medicine, and others, including alternative medicine. This selected inventory of exercises has been derived from many sources.

"STRETCH IT OUT"

Warm-ups and stretches have become the order of the day, whether preparing for an aerobics class, engaging in a competitive sport, doing a health club workout, or jogging. Gentle, repetitive, low-intensity activities are combined with stretching of muscles. This warms the muscles by increasing blood supply to them. Warm-ups also tend to increase the amount of fluid in joint cartilages, causing them to expand and helping to avoid joint injury during exercise and sports.

Applications of heat contribute to warming muscles.

Warm muscles can be stretched further without injury, and when they contract they can do more work with less chance of being injured. Weak, tight muscles are especially vulnerable to injury, whether in the back or elsewhere, and as previously described, back muscles are especially likely to fall into this category.

Stretching also increases the range of motion of a joint as well as increasing the blood supply to the muscle. It is also known to enhance body coordination and help develop a sense of body awareness. Body awareness means that you remain cognizant of where your body is in space, whether or not its alignment is appropriate, which muscles are tight and which are relaxed, and can perceive and respond to your body's level of comfort. Not least important is that stretching helps develop a personal sense of well-being and refreshment and is a useful tool in the management of stress.

Muscles are stretched slowly. No jerking or bouncing action should ever occur during stretching, or any other back exercise. If a muscle were to be stretched suddenly a protective reflex would be brought into play, a reflex that acts to shorten the muscle to prevent injury.

Stretching is done steadily, purposefully, to the point of gentle tension. Hold it for six, ten, or twelve seconds, depending on your preference, and then begin slowly to release the stretch for about the same number of seconds.

Accompany your stretch by breathing, which acts to support the benefits of the controlled stretch and subsequent muscle relaxation. Avoid shallow, jerky breathing. Improved breathing helps to slow down the stretch and assists in relaxing uninvolved muscles. Before the stretch take a deep breath and let it out. Then inhale as you stretch and exhale as you let go of the stretch. Finish with another relaxing breath.

Do your stretches while lying down, sitting, standing, kneeling, or even on all fours, the position in which you did the pelvic tilt on hands and knees. Stretches involving back arching, and therefore back muscle contraction, usually are done first in the horizontal position, or in the water where you are weightless, to minimize gravitational pulls on the structures of your lower back.

Stretches are offered in a suggested progression. Individual needs and preferences may take precedence.

1. Supine Body Stretch

While lying on your back with arms at your sides, draw up your knees with the soles of your feet flat and several inches apart. First, tilt your pelvis by slowly pressing the middle of your back into the bed as you have already done.

Then, following the above stretching guidelines, slowly inhale while bringing the middle of your back up and off the bed or mat to your point of comfort, hold for several seconds, and exhale while slowly letting your back sink again down to the bed.

If this feels good to your back, rest for several seconds and do one more. This time try it with your knees apart, still keeping your feet just inches apart.

At first it is not necessary that your back leave the floor. The goal is never to increase the arch beyond the shallowest of curves. In this stretch you are, for the first time, reversing the pelvic tilt as you tighten back muscles and stretch the muscles of your chest.

Finish with a pelvic tilt to help relax and stretch your back muscles.

2. Supine Total Body Stretch

While lying on your back with raised knees and tilted pelvis, raise your arms straight above your head against your ears, and slowly slide your heels down to straighten your legs while maintaining the pelvic tilt. Keep your toes pointed toward the ceiling. Release the tilt momentarily. Become aware of each muscle that is being stretched. Breathe and once again draw up your knees to release the stretch. If there is no room on the carpet or mat to raise your arms above your head, fold them above your head or extend them to the sides.

Try a variation on the theme: Again, slide both heels toward the foot of the bed, but this time attempt to stretch one heel slightly farther down than the other. This tilts the pelvis to the side. Draw it back to the level of the other heel and repeat with the opposite heel. This time keep the pelvic tilt throughout. Do this exercise with your arms at your sides.

This total body stretch can also be done in the water. The back arch can also be done in the water. First float on your back. Then drop your head back slightly in the water and let your legs drop.

3. Side-Lying Hip and Back Stretch

On your side with straight knees, draw up your top knee as far as you comfortably can and drop it onto the bed while keeping your bottom leg straight. Move your bottom leg back slightly for a minimal back arch. Do the stretch to your point of comfort. Then switch sides and repeat.

This is an exercise you may do almost automatically at intervals throughout the night when you need a stretch and change of position.

4. Rotation of Arms and Legs

While supine, keep your knees straight and slowly rotate them and your feet inward from the hip. Then, turning your knees outward, slowly rotate them outward to your point of comfort.

Do the same with your arms while keeping your elbows straight. Extend your fingers as you rotate both arms from the shoulders on their axis—

first inward, then outward. You can do this arm
stretch almost anytime during your day.

5. Ankle Circles

While supine, or sitting at your desk or in a
plane, flex your toes toward the ceiling, then extend them by pointing your toes. Circle them a few
times inward, then outward, causing your ankles
to rotate. The blood circulation in your legs often
needs this boost, and ankles support your body
weight.

6. Two Back Stretches

You have already done both of these, one as an
initial part of your back conditioning and the
other as a way of tying your shoes using proper
body mechanics. Note that in both your knees remain flexed.

The first is, while lying supine, to draw one or
both knees slowly up to your chest while maintaining your pelvic tilt and then release.

The second has already been suggested, and
it is an excellent way of relieving a tired back.
While sitting in a chair, lean forward over your
knees as if to pick up an object from the floor.
Another less convenient alternative is to kneel on
the floor with your forearms on the floor and your
head resting on your crossed arms.

There is a caveat: Do *not* sit on the floor with
straight legs and bend forward between your outstretched legs to stretch out your back. As you did
not stand and bend forward with straight knees,
do not sit and do this either. Although still frequently suggested by many sources, it is unnecessarily hard on the structures of your lower back
and can cause injury even to a problem-free back.
Instead, continue to do your back stretches with
bent knees.

7. Shoulder Circles

In the standing or sitting position bring your shoulders forward, rotate them up toward your ears, bring them back as far as you comfortably can, and then down in normal position. The motion is circular.

Rotate them in the opposite direction several times, and drop them down in a relaxed position. This exercise helps to relieve upper back muscle tension and reminds you not to hold your tension in your shoulders and neck. It is useful when you find yourself sitting or standing for prolonged periods.

A variation is simply to bring your shoulders up to your ears occasionally and then to drop them down into normal position.

8. Neck Stretches

Avoid neck circles because there is some potential for injury. The following is a better alternative to stretch your neck.

With shoulders dropped and level, raise your chin and gently let your head fall backward; hold for several seconds.

Return your head to normal position and then let it drop directly to the side, toward one dropped shoulder. Return to normal position and let it drop to the opposite side and then to normal position.

Finally, let it drop gently forward before returning to normal position. Take plenty of time for each position change.

Try something else. Elongate the back of your neck with your chin dropped down as though trying to make a double chin. Repeat, but this time when you drop your chin, drop it diagonally to the right. Try it again, dropping your chin to the left, and release.

9. Two Chest Stretches

When you arch your back, the result is stretching your chest muscles. The following give a more complete stretch. The first is performed in many Yoga classes.

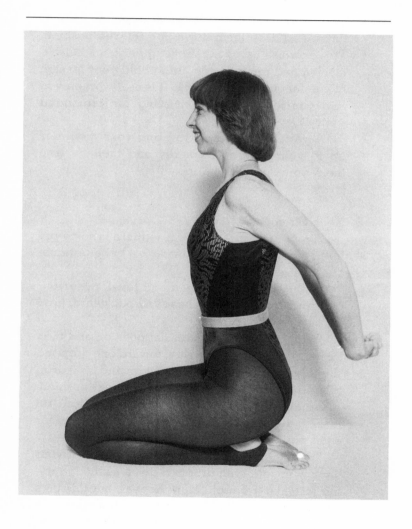

☐ Level Three. Kneeling Chest Stretch

Either standing or kneeling, clasp your hands behind your back with arms held straight behind you at hip level. Now, keeping your arms straight and your chin tilted upward, raise your hands, still clasped behind you, up toward the ceiling as high as you comfortably can. Your shoulders are pulled backward. Take a couple of deep, satisfying breaths, and enjoy.

There is another chest stretch that is easy to do in many circumstances throughout the day. Stand in the doorway with your hands at chest level and braced on the doorjambs on either side of you. With your feet stationary in the doorway, lean forward until you feel the stretch.

10. One More Back Stretch

This one starts like at least two of the Yoga postures but stops short of the possibility of placing body weight on the neck, especially the flexed neck. Many exercise physiology experts see this as an unnecessary risk.

On the bed, supine, draw up your knees and

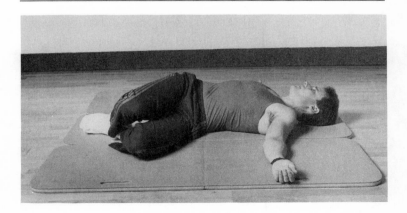

Level Three. Rotational Stretch

use your hands to brace your hips and raise them up and off the bed. Let your flexed knees and relaxed legs hang over your nose. You will feel a satisfying stretch in your entire back, and the gravitational change from the upright posture can be welcome.

11. Rotational Stretches

Place yourself supine with raised knees on a bed or a floor mat. Keeping your shoulders flat on the bed, slowly swing both knees to one side, raise them back to the midline, and then swing them toward the other side.

Try a variation: While supine with both knees raised and slightly apart, drop your right knee to the outside down to the bed. Then drop it to the left toward the floor but in the direction of your left leg. Do the same with your left leg.

Do another variation, in the water. As you swim, leading with your elbows and using your legs to assist you, rotate your body 180 degrees. Try it twisting once in each direction.

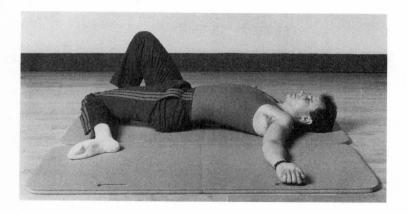

Level Three. Rotational Stretch, One Knee

12. Inner Thigh Stretch

Previous exercises done with knees apart have offered you the chance for inner thigh stretch. These stretches are important for proper bending and lifting, and they assist with postural balance.

It is more difficult to find exercises that strengthen these adductor muscles than it is to stretch them. Possibilities for strengthening include horseback riding and use of health club exercise equipment. One inner thigh exercise will be presented among the Level Three exercises.

Sit cross-legged in tailor position with your lower back supported with a pillow against the wall. For greater stretch (and this is also a Yoga posture) place the soles of your feet together and bring them toward your body as far as you comfortably can.

13. The Standing Squat

You have already done a squat in Level One while side-lying on the bed. The standing squat is performed, with knees somewhat apart, on your feet with your heels flat on the floor and toes pointed straight ahead or slightly outward. This stretch is not for everyone. Without practice it is difficult for many people. It places maximum flexion on the knees and maximum stretch on the back muscles, quadriceps, and calf muscles.

This is the position adopted frequently, for many tasks, by a large part of the world's population and is especially important in preparation for childbirth. It is the most physiologic position for the process of giving birth and is now used regularly in hospitals and birthing centers.

First stand, then drop down into the squat while keeping your back straight even as it inclines forward in the direction of your knees. You may need to balance yourself against a piece of furniture, and at first you may not be able to drop your heels onto the floor if your calf muscles have not been stretched.

14. Standing Side Stretches

Side stretches involve lateral flexion, and they stretch key postural muscles.

Stand with feet pointing straight ahead and slightly apart and arms at your sides. Do the pelvic tilt and slowly bend directly to the side, with no forward or backward bend. Hold for several seconds at your point of tension and return to the upright position. Repeat, stretching muscles on your opposite side.

You can increase the effectiveness of this exercise by raising your arm on the side being stretched. For example, as you bend to the right, curve your left arm up in the direction of your ear and over your head. The arm must stay in line with your body, neither forward nor backward.

15. Standing Trunk Rotation

With pelvis tilted, stand with shoulders slightly raised and at chin level. Slowly twist your body to one side. Return to center, then move toward the opposite side before again returning to center. Do not push your limit. Golf swings involve standing trunk rotation.

16. Standing Quad Stretch

Many athletic programs include this quad stretch, which can be done easily in many situations. Stand, grasp one foot, and then pull it directly up behind you in the direction of your buttocks. Use your other hand to balance yourself against a piece of furniture or the wall. While doing this do not bend forward.

Hold for several seconds while stretching to

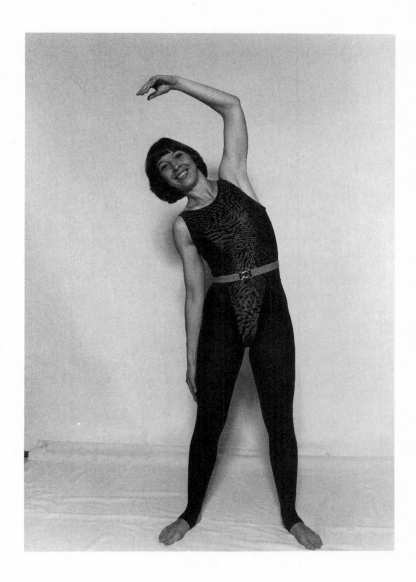

☐ Level Three. Standing Side Stretch

your point of comfort, then release. Do the same with the other leg.

For a less complete but often preferable standing quad stretch bend one knee, with heel pointed down, to the point of complete flexion, bringing

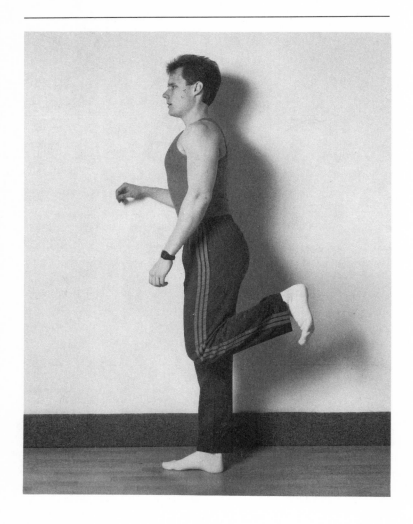

Level Three. Standing Quad Stretch

your heel up directly behind you. Lead with your heel. The difference in this stretch is that you are not using your hand to pull up your foot. This gives the quad stretch without overstressing the knee joint.

17. The Inverted "V"

Another exercise from the Yoga postures stretches your calves, the back of your legs, and your back. It also increases your "body awareness" when you try to figure out exactly what position your body is in! You may need a mirror at first!

Your body weight rests on your hands and your feet. Your buttocks form the top of the inverted "V." Your knees are straight (extended), as are your elbows. Your head is down in line with your shoulders and arms, neither raised nor dropped, to maintain the "V" alignment of your body. Your arms, head, and trunk form one part of the angle of the "V" and your legs form the other.

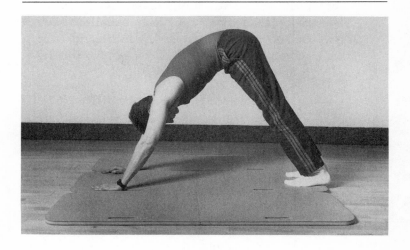

Level Three. Inverted "V" Back Stretch

"NOW DO YOUR BACK"

The muscle stretching you have just done increases the flexibility of joints and helps protect muscles against injury. Stretches usually precede strengthening exercises and are done before a sports activity. At the conclusion of an intense sports activity they become part of the cool-down.

Strengthening muscles serves to protect the body against physical harm. The stability of your joints depends on the dynamic muscular forces surrounding each joint. And the contractile power of your voluntary muscles is the source of your ability to propel your body, permitting you to move about your world.

1. Walking

   Walking for fifteen to thirty minutes with correct posture, including tightened abdomen, at least several times per week is an excellent back exercise. If you place your hands behind your waist as you walk you can feel some of the activity of your back muscles.

2. Prone Lying

   Lie prone on your abdomen for several seconds, or longer. Feel your back muscles contract. Bend your knees, bringing your heels toward your buttocks for a quad stretch. Then straighten your legs and spread them apart into a "V" on the carpet before bringing them back parallel.

   Turn over onto your side or back at the first sign of discomfort and tilt your pelvis to relieve any feelings of strain resulting from tightened back muscles in the prone position.

3. Bridging

On your back, supine, draw up your knees with the soles of your feet on the floor. Arch your back to your point of comfort, thereby contracting your back muscles to help lift your buttocks off the carpet or mat. Do the motion slowly and hold it for six, ten, or a dozen seconds, whatever feels best to you. Keep the time short, especially at first. Release.

Try it first with knees together. Then do it with knees apart. Do it with heels down, then try it with heels raised.

4. Standing Back Exercise

This exercise may remind you of ballet training. Many find this an exercise they like to do.

Stand with your left hand on a wall or with both hands on doorjambs to help maintain your balance. Raise your right leg behind you. Straighten your right knee and lead with your

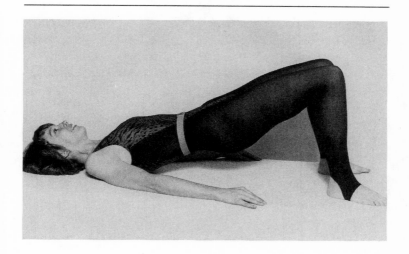

Level Three. Bridging

right heel as you raise the leg. Your foot is rotated to the right.

Swing your straightened right leg backward and diagonally to the right. Keep your body up-

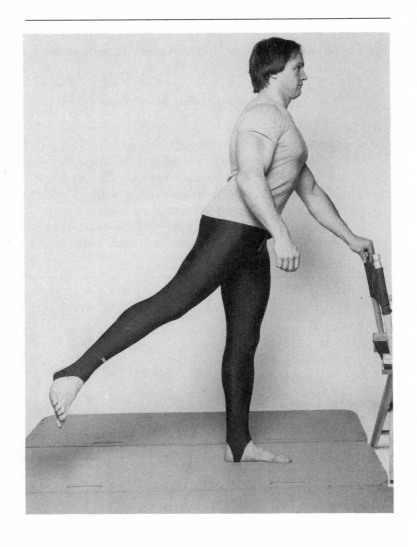

Level Three. Standing Back Exercise

right. Do not lean forward to make this exercise easier. Hold for several seconds. Note the contraction of your back and buttock muscles. Release. Repeat with the opposite leg.

Do the same exercise trying to swing your leg more backward than diagonally to increase the contraction of your back muscles. Note also the contraction of your hamstring muscles in the back of your legs. Here you are tightening, not stretching, your hamstrings and buttocks.

5. The Crawl Swimming Stroke

One reason swimming seems to help so many problem backs is that it requires shortening of back muscles, which strengthens them. If your head is raised up out of the water occasionally, instead of merely turned to the side, the contraction of back muscles is increased.

When swimming is accompanied by the straight leg kick the back muscles get more of a workout—too much at first for a weak or sore back. You can minimize the range or rate of kicking until you are certain that this will feel good to your back and will not irritate the lower back structures.

In the water, while you are both supine and prone, straight leg kicking has its place in a back strengthening program. First shorten your abdominal muscles and tighten your buttock muscles into the pelvic tilt.

While prone in the water, tilt your pelvis and spread your legs apart to form a "V." This contracts your hip muscles besides giving you another opportunity to stretch the inner thigh muscles.

6. The Breaststroke

This swimming stroke increases the arch of the back beyond that required by the crawlstroke. Do it only if it feels good to your back.

7. All Fours with Leg Extension

On your hands and knees, tilt your pelvis so that your back is straight, not sagging into an arch. Then, keeping your head in line with your body and your pelvis tilted, flex one knee and draw it toward your chest. Then extend that same leg directly backward in line with your body, straightening your knee and pointing your toe. Hold for several seconds and release. Repeat with the opposite leg.

Very little, if any, obvious arch in your back appears. Nevertheless, your back muscles are exercised, as are your abdominals, your hamstrings, and your arms, shoulders, and neck.

Do a variation: Extend the opposite arm forward at the same time that you extend one leg back. Your body is both stretched and strengthened.

The common error made is overly rapid repeti-

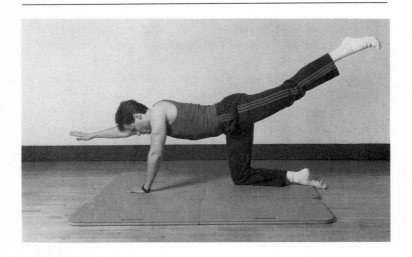

☐ Level Three. All Fours, Leg and Arm Extension

tions with backs alternately flexed and overly extended. The motion should be slow with no back
hyperextension. The focus remains on the pelvic
tilt.

8. Prone Head and Shoulder Raise
    Lie face down with your arms at your sides.
Attempt to raise your head and shoulders off the
carpet or floor mat. Depending on your back
strength and body type, the number of inches you
can come up will vary.
    The goal is not to increase the number of de-
grees you can raise your upper body, although
this proficiency does tend to increase. Hold only
for a few seconds before releasing. Doing it once
is enough. Then to release the tension in your
back muscles, turn onto your side and draw up
your knees or turn onto your back, either with
knees straight or bent, and do the pelvic tilt.
    Do not push yourself up off the floor with your
hands.

9. Prone Leg Raise
    While lying prone with head down, brace your

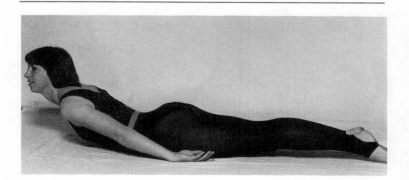

Level Three. Prone Head and Shoulder Raise

abdominal muscles, tighten your buttocks, and attempt to raise your extended legs several inches off the floor. Try it first with one leg only. Hold for a few seconds only before releasing. Turn over and do a pelvic tilt.

Repeat the exercise. This time after raising your extended legs off the mat or floor a couple of inches, turn your toes outward and spread your legs apart into a "V" as feels comfortable. Hold for two or three seconds before bringing the legs back parallel and allowing them to drop down onto the mat. Finish by turning over and gently bringing your knees to your chest for several seconds to rest your back.

In neither exercise 8 nor 9 should someone hold down your lower back while you raise either shoulders or legs, even if you see this suggestion in print.

10. The "Three Point" Exercise

Lie supine on a firm surface with your knees straight. Your arms remain at your sides, and there is no pillow under your head. Visualize this exercise in your mind before you try it.

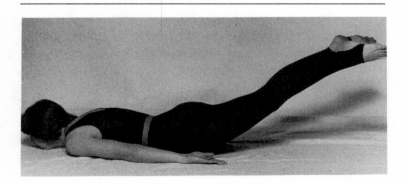

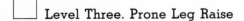 Level Three. Prone Leg Raise

Arch your back minimally. Then tighten your buttocks and leg muscles. Your goal is to support your entire body on your shoulders and heels. Hold for six seconds, or less at first, and release. Turn onto your side to relax your back. Finish with a pelvic tilt to increase back comfort.

At first this back strengthening exercise may sound impossibly difficult, but for a fit and healthy back an occasional try at this can feel good. If you are overweight, have generally poor body fitness, an unresolved structural problem in your back, or back muscles already contracted into painful spasm, this exercise is not for you. If in doubt, consult with your medical practitioner.

However, this "three point" exercise can help your back and is in every way preferable to the traditional push-up, which places, in the prone attitude, body weight on hands and toes. The push-up is very hard on the joints of the back and provides no benefit that cannot be obtained in more desirable ways despite its continued popularity in many organized sports programs. The traditional push-up was not designed as a back exercise.

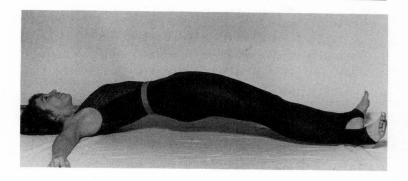

Level Three. "Three Point" Exercise

"THE LEGBONE IS CONNECTED TO THE THIGHBONE"

Several exercises in Level Three add to "the icing on the cake." They permit you to strengthen other muscles that add to back fitness. For example, you have vertical abdominal muscles, but you also have abdominal muscles that are angled to the side, called the obliques. Another simple exercise adds to the strength of your hip muscles. Additional shoulder and upper back strength helps, too.

Try the following:

1. Diagonal Sit-ups
     Lie on your back with raised knees and arms crossed on your chest. Tighten your abdomen. Pull your head and shoulders up off the floor, aiming your right elbow toward your left knee. Do this several times; then repeat, this time bringing your left elbow toward your right knee. Repeat.

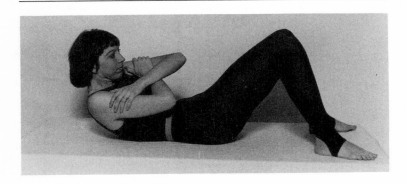

Level Three. Diagonal Sit-up

Although abdominal weakness tends to be concentrated in the vertical-running muscles with the greatest weakness in the midline, it also helps to strengthen the obliques for a stronger body.

To increase the difficulty of the exercise, place your arms behind your head. Raise your head and shoulders, bringing each elbow toward the opposite knee. Do *not* use your crossed arms behind your head to pull your neck forward, producing possible neck strain.

2. Diagonal Curl-ups

This is the same as above, but drawing both shoulders and knees off the floor, again drawing right shoulder toward left knee and vice versa.

3. The Buttock Walk

You will feel the active muscles in this exercise. Sit on the floor with your legs flexed and soles of your feet on the floor. Bring your left

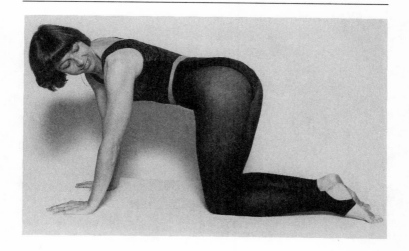

☐ Level Three. Wagging Your Tail

buttock forward, followed by your right buttock, and then your left buttock. Yes, you really can walk on your buttocks!

4. Wagging Your Tail

This exercise is for your waistline. In the all-fours position draw in your abdominal muscles to assume the pelvic tilt. Slowly twist your upper body to the right, as if to look at your tailbone while bringing your lower back also to your right. Repeat, this time turning to the left.

5. Modified Push-ups

On hands and knees, drop your nose to the floor and push back up. Your back is most protected if your knees remain under your hips instead of back of your hips. This exercise benefits arms and shoulders.

True, this is not the way to develop maximum arm and shoulder strength, but there are other ways to do this, including the use of weights under trained supervision.

6. Sculling in the Water

You can gain a modicum of upper body strength by sweeping both arms simultaneously

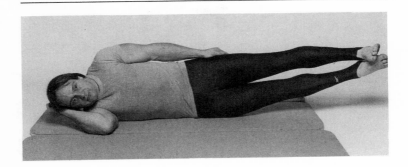

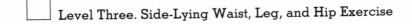
Level Three. Side-Lying Waist, Leg, and Hip Exercise

through the water on your back. Bring both arms up over your ears above your head and pull yourself through the water.

7. Inner Thigh Tightening

Lie on your side and cross your top leg over to rest your knee on the bed as you have already done during the third stretching exercise. Now raise your straightened bottom leg up toward the ceiling. At first you may have difficulty raising it more than an inch or two. Feel the pull on the adductor muscle of your inner thigh. Lie on your other side and do the same for your other thigh.

8. One More Good Side-Lying Exercise for Waist, Legs, and Hips

This exercise helps protect your back. Lie on your side, tilt your pelvis, and straighten both legs. Raise your top leg toward the ceiling, keeping it directly over the other leg, neither forward nor backward, as far as you comfortably can. Lower it so that it rests atop the bottom leg once more.

Now *raise both legs toward the ceiling.* You will be using different muscles in each leg to hoist your legs against gravity. Note in which muscles you feel the pull.

Switch to your other side, straighten both legs, and tighten your abdominal muscles. Keep your legs together, straight, and directly in line with your body. Raise them once again in the direction of the ceiling.

A WORD ON SEX AND YOUR BACK

A number of previous books (see Bibliography) have offered advice on sex and the "bad" back. Suggested positions for sex may or may not work for couples. Proffered suggestions regarding sex have even included the comment that if the pleasure exceeds the pain, then go right ahead. Many will disagree, particularly when this comment is made with the concurrent admonition contained in all the literature to do nothing that causes pain.

Strained backs have occurred during sexual activity. This is most likely when the back has been overly arched, known as hyperextension.

Recently there have been interesting comments that you might wish to consider for better understanding of your back. When sexual activity involves assuming the pelvic tilt, combined with a moderate degree of back extension, a pelvic rock is done as the pelvis is "rocked" through its range of motion. Flexibility of the spine is involved with the pelvic tilt alternating with moderate back arching. Abdominal and back strengthening can occur. Sexual activity utilizing the back's normal range of motion can help to prevent back problems.

The conclusion can only be that, for a fundamentally problem-free back, sexual activity is a beneficial back exercise. For a weak, tight back, in fact, sex becomes one of your better back exercises.

CHAPTER NINE
WOULD A HEALTH CLUB HELP?

$\square$

During the 1970s new exercise equipment became increasingly available. By the 1980s health clubs began to proliferate in many settings, in neighborhoods, shopping malls, schools, and corporate environments. Publicity about the crucial role of exercise in maintaining health, and even longevity, sparked public interest.

At first the goal of many club members was limited largely to assistance in weight loss along with the opportunity for socializing. Others joined for specific training in lifting weights. For some, body shaping through muscle strengthening and the resulting muscle definition has been the motivating force.

Cardiovascular fitness centers are included in many health clubs, and aerobic classes for cardiovascular conditioning are an important part of health club programs. All age groups are welcome. The knowledgeable older population, along with younger groups, is especially aware of the necessary emphasis placed on the importance of cardiovascular conditioning.

Health clubs are still a place of mystery for many. What is the equipment's purpose, and how is it used? Could an injury occur? What clothes does one wear? How often does one come? Even, where does one put one's coat? Some who join are making a commitment to an unknown. At first view it is obvious that there are many opportunities for exercise, all of them concentrated in one location, the health club.

In general, health clubs have not promoted themselves as sources of help for a "bad" back, nor specifically as sources of back protection and prevention of back problems. In fact, people with back problems tend to avoid health clubs just because they do have problem backs. However, health clubs, wisely used, can help your back. If you choose, you can use the available exercise equipment to maximize your back fitness. One of the machines is specifically designed to strengthen back muscles.

The health club activities complement what you have already learned. But sometimes, for example, the abdominal muscle strengthening done at the club can replace the abdominal exercises you do at home. Aerobic classes, however, do not replace back exercises. Participation in these classes will be safer if you have already attained your goal of a fit back.

Most clubs cannot, economically, offer the full range of fitness equipment and activities unless their space is ample and their membership large. They may have a pool, sauna, whirlpool, juice bar, tennis courts, squash or racketball courts, and basketball courts. Club members may use the showers and locker rooms. All clubs will provide a tour of their facilities before you join.

You will find several types of exercise machines, each designed to strengthen a particular muscle group. These may be arranged in a sequence and called a "circuit." There will also be free weights for lifting. Use these only under supervision of a fitness instructor.

Aerobic conditioning equipment also strengthens muscles. You may discover rowing machines, cross country skiing machines, stationary bicycles, walking or jogging machines, and stair-climbing machines. Yes, you can climb fifty flights of stairs while your heart rate is continuously monitored and your rate of climb and caloric expenditure are recorded on a screen!

One or more fitness instructors are available at all times. Ask about their credentials and experience. Some have degrees in exercise physiology. They may be certified by the American College of Sports Medicine. You need close supervision, especially at the beginning, even to ride the stationary bicycle. For example, is the seat height adjusted correctly? Is your back straight? How fast and for how long should you pump? Are you taking your heart rate by placing your fingers on the artery of your neck? What is the "target" heart rate for your age?

The rowing machines appear simple, but the types vary. What load should you select? Is your technique correct? Are you avoiding back arching as you pull back on the "oars"? Again, what is your target heart rate, and how long should you maintain it? Are you doing warm-ups and cool-downs? How frequently should you "row"?

Target heart rates are determined by subtracting your age from the number 220. Then figure 70 percent of this number. Next, figure 85 percent of this number. The range between these two numbers is the training zone for your aerobic exercise workout. For example, if you are sixty-five your minimum heart rate will be 109. If you are thirty-five it will be 130, and if you are twenty it will be 140. Keep the heart rate below the maximum for your age group. Most clubs have a chart with this information posted on the wall.

Health clubs require prepayment for three months to a year. Sometimes there are special introductory offers. The club is then yours to use as frequently and extensively as you wish. Choosing a convenient location—for example, on the way home from work—may be more important than joining a more distant club with a wider selection of equipment.

Among the motivations to continue is the feedback you obtain on your progress in terms of lowered heart rate, increased exercise time, increased muscle strength as measured by added weights on the machines, and more enjoyment of the activities. Body weight may decrease, if this is what you wish, but it may not, even though you feel thinner and some body measurements have decreased. Although the amount of fat may be less, the amount of muscle mass may increase. Muscle weighs more than fat.

Exercise increases the production of brain chemicals known as endorphins, which promote a sense of well-being. This change in brain chemistry is thought to be one reason why those who are accustomed to physical exercise often feel anxious and deprived if they cannot continue to be active.

DOING THE CIRCUIT

Exercise machines of any type or brand help you to isolate, identify, and know your muscles. You already know the names of muscles most important to acquiring a fit back, but the circuit puts you in touch with a few others as well. The machines allow you to strengthen many muscle groups from your neck to your ankles, opportunities difficult to duplicate in the daily lives of most.

The machines provide what is called a high-intensity exercise. During ordinary daily activity, only some, not all, muscle fibers of a muscle are "fired" by nerve impulses, because the muscle is not being worked to capacity. The machine brings each muscle group through the entire range from full stretch to complete contraction. The maximum possible muscle fibers of each muscle group are used. The performance may or may not be repeated to the point where it is difficult to perform another repetition without a period of rest. Perhaps you can move the weight six times but not a dozen times.

The repetitions are both brief and infrequent. The suggested number of repetitions may be approximately eight. Do the first two or three repetitions very slowly for a warm-up. Then about two seconds may be needed for the contraction. Four seconds may be suggested for the release. A slow release is considered very important. All motions are done smoothly. Do not hold your breath, and try to relax uninvolved muscles.

At least a forty-eight-hour interval should elapse before the machine is used again. Muscle strengthening takes place a day or two after your workout. Aerobic exercise is also done two or three times per week. Aerobics classes, if taken more than three times per week, have been shown to increase the possibility of injury.

When you come to the club, plan to do the entire circuit, not your abdominals and neck one day and your back and hips another, but use no more than a dozen machines on any one day. You can see that the training is intense and brief. The body functions best when worked in its entirety and is then rested in entirety. But you can skip two or three of the machines as you prefer or as your needs seem to indicate.

When you can do a dozen or so repetitions, the resistance is increased. Equipment may vary, and you should continue to consult with your fitness instructor. Start with the lowest possible resistance until you understand the machine and know what you can do. Keep written records.

Many of the machines have seat belts to help protect your back. For many of the machines, it is important first to tighten your abdomen to assume the pelvic tilt. There are also numbered seat adjustments for proper body alignment. The fitness instructor will suggest the correct position for you. By making a note of these you will know the position when you come back to that machine. Also, written directions beside each machine often summarize proper technique. They also inform you which muscles are being worked when you use that machine.

Meet a few more of your muscles that are involved in developing a strong back.

1. Besides the erector spinae muscles, which, when contracted, arch your back, you have the trapezius muscle, a flat, triangular muscle. It extends from the base of your skull, across both shoulders, and comes to a point halfway down the spinal column. It is involved in posture and in back strength.

2. The latissimus dorsi of your upper back are large muscles on each side of the spine that run somewhat crosswise on your back. They, too, are involved in upper back strength and help define the shape of your back.

3. The deltoid muscle is draped over the top of each shoulder and allows you to move your arm forward, to the side, and backward.

4. The buttock muscle is the gluteus maximus, but there are other gluteal muscles, the gluteus medius and the gluteus minimus, which are on the outside of the hipbone. These two muscles allow you to spread your thighs apart. This is called hip abduction. The iliopsoas are the frontal hip muscles that allow you to bring your thighs forward.

5. Your pectoral muscles in the front of your chest allow you to pull your arms down and across your torso. They are involved in posture and help to define body shape.

6. Your calf muscle, which when adequately stretched helps you to stand with correct body alignment, is called the gastrocnemius muscle.

7. A review of the muscles of your upper leg reminds you that when you lie prone or stand, the hamstrings bend your legs. When you sit, the quadriceps act to straighten your legs. The inner thigh adductors allow you to bring your legs together. Strong thigh muscles help to stabilize the otherwise easily injured knee joint, although knee problems affect the back only indirectly. The circuits have machines for each of these muscles. With each machine a part of your body—in this case, your legs—moves in a predetermined track. The proper development of upper leg muscles can improve the appearance of your thighs.

When you use the machines, the following occurs: While prone, you flex your legs against resistance (hamstrings). While seated, you straighten your legs against resistance (quadriceps). While seated, you bring your separated, straightened legs together against a measured amount of resistance (adductors). While seated with extended legs parallel, you separate your legs against measured resistance (hip abduction). As the weeks pass and the motion becomes so easy that the resistance is just not enough, you add another weight.

The exercise machine circuits include equipment that strengthens the abdominal muscles, both the vertical recti and the obliques, and equipment that strengthens the back. When using the latter machine for strengthening the erector spinae, in which you try to lean back against resistance, the weights must be increased only gradually, and the back must not arch. Start with lowest weights for the erector spinae of your back. It is easy to overload these muscles without realizing it.

When using free weights, the bench presses are safest for your back. Because you lift while on your back there is no compression loading on your spine. For weight lifting make sure you obtain individual coaching and that motions are as smooth as possible. In positions where there is vertical spine pressure use a wide belt to help protect your lower back against the forces of compression.

GAME PLAN

The two secrets to safe sports are preparatory body conditioning and the use of proper techniques. Sports can help to strengthen your back and improve overall body conditioning. Some sports require an already strong back as a prerequisite to the safety of the sport, as in contact sports. There is also the popular concept of the risks faced by "the weekend athlete" where conditioning, and perhaps techniques, too, may be deficient.

White (see Bibliography) states the important fact that cumulative sports injuries may occur until a disc, ligament, or bone fails. He goes on to discuss the problems with lifting and twisting, as in a ballet sequence where the male partner must lift the female, and the risks of football tackling and wrestling matches. The result may be arthritis of the joints, fatigue fractures of spinal bones, or vertebral injuries to the projections (facet joints) in back of the spinal bones associated with concomitant back arching and lifting.

His encouragement to engage in the sport even if some muscle aches or residual sensations do occur may be beneficial if only to emphasize the point that lack of exercise has a strong correlation with back problems. Generally, those who have experienced a "bad" back hardly dared to move, avoiding exercise as they might the plague.

Mild muscle aches the following day, especially in

legs or shoulders, may be part of the conditioning, not indications to halt the activity. Pain is another story. Often only you, knowing how you feel, can decide what, how often, and how much.

When enjoying your sport or sports (1) keep in mind the principles you have learned about stretching, bending, and lifting; (2) make the conditioning described in Levels One, Two, and Three back exercises an important part of your self-care; and (3) analyze the required motions of the sport in the light of what you have learned about back protection.

The following comments are offered on a number of common sports. The benefits of walking and swimming have already been discussed.

1. Jogging

   Proper fit and padding of shoes, the running surface, the body weight of the runner, and the smoothness of the gait are important considerations according to some studies. The increased miles run per week correlate with the increased possibility of injury to back, hip, knee, ankle, or foot. Consult with athletic trainers or fitness instructors. Some runners do cross training, meaning that on some days they substitute another aerobic activity for long-distance jogging.

   Jogging does not act to strengthen back and abdominal muscles, although it may appear to do so. Exercises for these muscles should be done as accompaniments to jogging.

2. Tennis

   The sudden motions and the twists involved may be hard on a weak, tight back, but a fit back is good protection. Draw in the abdominals occasionally, and do not allow your back to sink into the swayback position.

3. Bicycling

Proper seat height without the need for excessive leg extension to pump the pedals is needed. Keep your back straight, not excessively curved outward into a "C" nor arched, whether using a ten-speed, which places more of your weight on arms and shoulders, or an English bike. Avoid impact injuries as a result of traffic, road obstructions, and sandy or rocky road edges.

Bicycling is often used to replace some jogging workouts, substituting activity that jars the spine, knees, and ankles with another high-intensity aerobic activity with a smoother motion.

4. Horseback Riding

Horseback riding can strengthen your back, abdomen, and thighs. However, the posting done while trotting, or trotting without posting, as in western-style riding, can be jarring on your back. So can jumping. Impact injuries are possible.

5. Basketball

As with tennis, there are quick motions and turns. Sudden impacts and falls can occur. Back fitness can help to prevent back injury.

6. Golf

Golf involves forward bending, twisting (rotation) of the body with feet in a fixed position, combined with the minor impact of the club against the ball. Fortunately, there is some flexion in the knees. A fit back is a protection against injury, and doing the pelvic tilt helps. Obviously, more knee flexion, a tight abdomen, and the least possible forward bend are best for your back.

7. Bowling

Bowling can be hard on a weak back, although it may not appear so. The lower back and hamstrings must be able to stretch. When bowling, the knees are turned slightly to the side away from the arm, which is releasing the ball, resulting in a slight body twist. Also, the late release of the ball brings the weight of the ball far from the body, as in a lever, placing demands on the shoulder and back. Focus on trying to reduce the degree of twist and keeping the abdomen tight.

8. Baseball

For pitchers, the techniques used vary. Unnecessary back arching can be avoided. Overuse injuries may occur.

For batters, as with golfers, there is a body twist with feet in a fixed position. There is a forward bend and also a substantial impact as the bat connects with the ball. The protection is a fit back, a straight back with knees flexed, and the pelvis tilted.

9. Skiing

Here the leg muscles take much of the impact, and the knees are flexed. The pelvic tilt continues to help. Good instruction and the attempt to fall correctly are essential for safety. Skiing is an excellent sport for body strengthening and conditioning. Choose skiing locations and conditions wisely to minimize the possibility of accidents and collisions.

10. Sailing

Be alert to the position in which you are holding your body. Sudden position changes may be required. If you sit with rigidly extended (straight) legs, especially with a rounded lower back, or with shoulders hunched forward, you are doing your back, even a fit back, no favor.

11. Rowing

When you tighten your abdomen and pull on both oars with a straight back, neither arched nor excessively rounded, rowing is an excellent conditioning and body strengthening exercise. Flexed knees help protect your back.

On the other hand, if in crew training you row with both hands on one oar, instead of sculling, in which you use two oars, the unbalanced forces on your back can result in backache even for a fit back.

12. Diving

The moderate back arch involved in most diving could be included in the section on back exercises. However, improper technique, or the use of sudden, alternating flexion and hyperextension, or sudden twists, can overstress your back. Landing in the water flat, or nearly so, on your back or stomach produces a jarring impact.

CHAPTER TEN
PREGNANCY AND AFTERWARD

□

Pregnancy and its associated back problems are legendary. They are almost seen as so "normal" that there are few referrals of pregnant women to orthopedists. Prenatal visits to the obstetrician are not particularly geared to dealing with backache, nor is a postnatal visit focused on getting into shape and preventing postnatal backaches.

Childbirth classes include back care, but most couples attend classes only when the pregnancy is well advanced, in the sixth or seventh month. During the six to eight sessions several suggestions are made for back comfort during pregnancy, but the special interest of the couples is directed toward the management of possible back pain in labor and preparing for labor, birth, and breast-feeding. Time is limited for imparting back care information.

At times community groups such as the "Y" or childbirth education associations offer pregnancy exercise classes. Postnatal classes may be available, too. Early in pregnancy many women express the need to know what exercises they should be doing, wondering, too, how to recover physically after the baby arrives.

Back care, including back exercises, is not markedly different during and immediately after pregnancy than at other times. There are modifications and a few exercises that are of particular importance. In previous pages I have alluded to the value of practicing squatting during pregnancy in preparation for delivery and to the desirability of limiting back extension exercises during pregnancy.

There are several especially valuable exercises, and none of them is new. All have been described in Levels One, Two, or Three, and most of those included below have for years been part of preparing for childbirth. The bridging exercise described in Level Three can be included if you wish.

EXPECTING AND EXERCISING

During early pregnancy the frequent nausea and fatigue of the first trimester may discourage a normally active life-style. During late pregnancy the enlarged abdomen may do the same, although possible backaches and swollen legs bring "what to do" questions from pregnant women.

The relaxin hormone from the pituitary gland circulates in the blood during pregnancy, its effects being to relax ligaments and joints. The tailbone, usually quite rigid in its position, can move slightly to enlarge the space in the pelvis. The pubic symphysis in the front of the pelvis is a fixed joint formed by two bones coming together, separated by fibrous cartilage. The effect of the relaxin allows these bones to separate enough to enlarge the pelvic area space. The rib cage may expand slightly. To some degree relaxin affects the soft tissues also, allowing them to stretch for childbirth. Its production stops at the time of birth, and the changes it caused are reversed.

During late pregnancy the hormone's effects often result in temporary discomfort in the pubic area and enough instability of that joint to cause the "waddle" gait of some women. Some women note occasional discomfort in ligaments supporting the uterus and in the rib area where abdominal muscles attach. Most of the discomfort, including backache, can be alleviated by postural accommodation and mild exercises.

Aerobic exercise can be continued during pregnancy, with the activity level reduced and partly dependent on the previous level of muscular strength and aerobic fitness. Bouncing activities always pose injury possibilities and are not recommended during pregnancy, nor those that could cause falls and accompanying impact injury. Jogging and many aerobic classes add stress to joints and ligaments, including those of the back, already less stable because of the aforementioned hormonal change. Fatigue should be avoided. Swimming, brisk walking, and sometimes bicycling are the favorite aerobic exercises during pregnancy.

During pregnancy dehydration is possible during aerobic exercise. Drink water frequently, even if thirst is not noted. Another concern is the need to avoid exercise of such high intensity that there could be oxygen deprivation to the baby or even excessively high body heat. Stop long before experiencing feelings of exhaustion, weakness, or dizziness, or excessive sweating. Hot tubs and whirlpools should not be used during pregnancy. They can produce excessive body heat or increased blood flow to the body surface, with the consequent risk of depriving oxygen-carrying blood to the placenta, through which nutrients and oxygen pass to the baby.

Abdominal muscle tightening exercises should be limited during pregnancy to avoid separation of the vertical abdominal muscles and consequent weakening of muscle support. Do not do the bent-knee sit-ups or curl-ups of Level Two nor the diagonal sit-ups of Level Three. A milder abdominal exercise is presented instead.

Do not bend your back forward over straight knees whether standing or sitting on the floor, pregnant or not. The same warnings on straight leg lifts in the supine position given elsewhere in this book apply even more strongly to pregnant women.

Avoid prolonged standing, which encourages painful back arching, overstretched abdominals, and the risk of fluid collection in legs and feet. Avoid prolonged sitting, which places stress on the spine and tends to weaken abdominal muscles. Position changes also encourage improved blood circulation. This is always so, pregnant or not, but is more significant during pregnancy. While sitting do ankle circles to aid circulation. Shoulder circles help circulation and ease strain in the upper back.

Exercises developed to ease the process of childbirth are remarkably similar to those that protect the back, a fact noted long ago. During pregnancy the pelvic tilt is indispensable to back comfort, requiring the continued practice of mild abdominal exercises. The hamstring muscles and those of the inner thigh must be stretched for proper bending and lifting as well as for birth. The pelvic floor (Kegel) exercise taught in Level Two is especially necessary during pregnancy to support the increased weight of the uterus. Strong thigh and buttock muscles also help to support increased abdominal weight.

During pregnancy do the following at least once each day. Preferably do several repetitions, either all at once or at a later interval. Also, find a time to rest during the day, if only briefly.

1. **Relieve body tension by doing the progressive relaxation of Level One.**

2. **Sit cross-legged on the floor for a lower back and inner thigh muscle stretch. Do not extend your legs in front of you.**

3. The pelvic rock exercise on all fours (Level One) stretches the back and tightens the abdomen. For a flexible spine, gently alternate pelvic tilt with mild back extension (arching) motion. The pelvic rock was discussed in the section on sex and your back.

Repeat several times the tilt, the arch, and again the tilt. The pelvic rock is an essential part of all childbirth classes. Start it early in pregnancy and use it for comfort during labor.

The all-fours position takes the weight of the baby off your spine during late pregnancy and may help in correct positioning of the baby for delivery.

4. On your back with raised knees do the pelvic tilt in the supine position (Level One) by pressing the middle of your back against the floor or exercise mat. Then tighten your buttocks before releasing. Repeat with knees apart.

During late pregnancy limit your time flat on your back because the weight of the uterus on a major blood vessel tends to reduce blood circulation to the baby. Do not sleep on your back during late pregnancy. Most women in advanced pregnancy are not comfortable for long on their backs anyway. Sleep on your side, perhaps with a thin pillow between your knees for back and hip comfort.

5. While lying on your side, arch your back slightly to stretch your chest and contract your back muscles. The crawl swimming stroke helps to strengthen your back.

6. While standing, tilt your pelvis to the side by shifting position from one straightened leg to the other and back again.

7. For strengthening the quadriceps, do a wall slide (Level Two) and hold for several seconds.

8. Additional suggestions include (a) the all-fours with leg extension of Level Three and (b) the modified push-up, also in Level Three and done on all fours.

9. Especially during pregnancy, walk with your pelvis tilted, your rib cage raised, the back of your neck stretched, and your chin level.

POSTPARTUM, BACK IN SHAPE

The malaise of early pregnancy is replaced by the heavier abdomen and returning energy of later pregnancy, to be followed by the excitement, fatigue, and added responsibilities of having the new family member. For each of these there are motivations to exercise, whether to remain in reasonable shape and physically fit, to do it for the baby, to relieve possible back discomforts of late pregnancy, or for an easier delivery.

After the baby is born, many women need only look in the mirror to find a reason, but appearance is not the only concern. It is even possible to pop a disc if the need for back care remains unacknowledged.

Available time is limited due to the near-constant infant needs during its first weeks. With the night demands of the baby taking their toll on daytime energy levels, added rest or sleep during the day becomes a must when the woman is at home. She may take the baby onto the sofa or bed to make life easier. Some of the exercises may be done in bed also. With a stronger abdomen and back the daily tasks will become less tiring.

Not everyone has a noticeably protruding abdomen after pregnancy. This good fortune may or may not result from exercise and muscle strengthening. It should not be due to limiting calories, because a weight gain of at least twenty-five pounds is now encouraged for a healthier baby. Good postural alignment starting immediately after childbirth, even on the same day, can affect appearance and, by working to assume the pelvic tilt and lift the rib cage, the muscle strengthening process already begins.

A protruding postpartum abdomen is not usually the result of a still-enlarged uterus. The uterus has shrunk to the size of a grapefruit within minutes of birth, and within days has virtually returned to its prepregnant size of a pear. Nursing the baby results in faster return to normal size because of the pituitary hormone released during the process of breast-feeding.

Extra pounds are usually not a substantial cause for a protruding abdomen. In any case, weight loss after childbirth is not a goal as long as the source of calories is nourishing food. Nutrients and calories are needed by the breast-feeding baby, helping possible extra fat to disappear. The nursing baby uses several hundred calories a day. The bottom line is that the problem of the protruding abdomen must be resolved by tightening the abdominal muscles that have been so greatly stretched during pregnancy.

CESAREAN BIRTH

Since approximately 1980 nearly a quarter of all births in the United States have been Cesarean births despite the continuing questions and concerns of consumer groups and of many professionals as well. Among the large numbers of those who have had Cesareans it has become clear that these women are not "exempt" from postpartum exercise. They are on their feet, usually within hours after birth, when anesthesia has worn off. This helps to avoid the possibility of incurring postoperative blood clots after days of unnecessary inactivity.

Soon after anesthesia has worn off the abdominals are

drawn in, sometimes using a pillow held firmly against the abdomen, at first to assist flattening and to help avoid incision pain. The tendency to hunch over in an attempt to avoid possible resulting incision pain must be resisted and, as always, the posture for standing and walking is the tilted pelvis and the lifted rib cage.

Some exercises, such as the curl-up and bent-knee sit-up, may be delayed for several weeks or longer, depending on the woman, how she feels, and her recovery from surgery. These are never the first exercises done after childbirth, whether Cesarean or not.

POSTPARTUM EXERCISES

After childbirth do the following exercises in the suggested order, increasing the difficulty over several weeks or more:

1. The Kegel pelvic floor exercises can be started right after birth, whether or not an incision (episiotomy) has been done to enlarge the vaginal opening. Drawing in these muscles helps support the organs in the pelvis and indirectly helps avoid backache.

2. Shortly after birth, even with the baby still resting against the mother's abdomen, she can begin gently to draw in the abdominals. This assumes the use of no regional anesthesia such as a spinal or epidural, which numbs and sometimes temporarily paralyzes the lower half of the body.

3. Walking, whether ten minutes or two or three hours after birth has occurred, is done using, as always, the pelvic tilt with raised rib cage.

4. While lying supine on the bed, raise knees and

head, checking for abdominal muscle separation as described in Level One. Use both hands to press the muscles toward the midline as though to reduce the separation and tighten the abdominals. Remember, some separation is to be expected.

5. While supine with your raised knees and the soles of your feet on the bed, swing your knees slowly to one side and then the other.

6. Do the pelvic rock on all fours as in Level One and as done during pregnancy. Begin within a few days of birth.

7. Do the pelvic rock in another position, on your back with bent knees. Tighten your abdomen for the tilt, release into a slight back arch, and then rock the pelvis again into the tilt.

    Straighten (extend) your legs while supine and again do the pelvic rock, moving the pelvis into the tilted position and then slightly arching your back, then return to the pelvic tilt. Extending the legs increases the difficulty of doing the pelvic tilt and rocking the pelvis.

8. While standing, do the pelvic tilt to the side by keeping your legs straight and raising first one hip, then the other. Buttocks are tucked under in the pelvic tilt. This is a waist exercise. It is done during pregnancy and is a useful one to continue.

9. Do the wall slides of Level Two for upper leg strengthening (quadriceps).

10. Tighten the abdomen and buttocks before doing curl-ups as in Level Two. Several weeks may be required before you try this. First work on the preceding exercises.

    The abdominal tightening is needed for full postpartum recovery even if it is not started for two or three months.

11. Tighten the abdomen before trying bent-knee sit-ups. When you are comfortable with these, do the diagonal curl-ups and diagonal sit-ups of Level Three.

12. Finally, start back extension exercises, doing the easy ones first. You have probably already tried the prone position shortly after birth in relief at being able once more to lie comfortably on your abdomen.

   The prone position is a good one to use right after delivery. It encourages good position of the uterus and helps to relieve "after pains" common to those who have borne two or more children, as the uterus returns to normal size.

13. If aerobic exercise classes are a favorite activity, be conservative and wait until you are sure that you are more than ready for them and are comfortable with the preceding exercises.

   If you bring your baby with you to the aerobics classes, be aware that the music in many of these classes is loud enough to produce possible hearing loss. If you have any doubts about the volume, ask the instructor to turn it down.

   After childbirth the first aerobic exercises are walking, swimming, and bicycling.

Most women now return home from the hospital on the third day after delivery, and often sooner from hospitals or midwife-staffed birthing centers. Therefore, the value of correct bending and lifting techniques cannot be overestimated.

During the early days, when the woman's abdominal muscles tend to sag and joints may still not have entirely regained their former stability, shopping, vacuuming, and prolonged standing in the kitchen should be done by her spouse or a friend. The priorities for women are the care of the baby, extra rest, top-quality nutrition, and muscle strengthening exercises. The early ones can be done while resting in bed. Part of the postpartum fatigue, and the possible backaches, are due to weakened muscles; household activities, however numerous, will not substitute for proper exercises.

As the baby grows, use a back carrier to transport him or her to ease back strain.

CHAPTER ELEVEN

MEDICINE AND YOUR BACK

For most backaches, as you now know, both the prevention and the treatment are largely up to you. Even if you should require major back surgery, much of the rehabilitation is dependent on you. Body positioning for bending and lifting, and the exercises that will protect your back in the future can be done only by you. Surgery does not mean that you never need do another thing for your back. In fact, the truth is quite the opposite.

Sometimes backs require medical care. There are illnesses, diseases, and disabilities that seriously challenge both the back sufferer's intelligence and persistence as well as the varied and ever-changing tools of the world of medicine. For the back patient there are descriptions in the literature of possible problems, but few resources on where to go, what might be done, or how to assess possible recommendations.

Individual situations vary, as do medical resources and medical opinions. Back patients often express the feeling of being in limbo, not knowing what or whom to trust, and uncertain of the questions to be asked. They suffer from both confusion and their chronic pain and disability.

There can be few absolutes, but back patients can have guidelines to assist them in obtaining a diagnosis of their problem or problems and to help them decide on a possible course of action, including the choice of medical care. An introduction to this topic was offered in the first chapter and also in the chapter on possible causes of back pain.

INDICATIONS FOR SEEKING MEDICAL CARE

Patients in obvious pain often appear at doctors' offices almost apologetically, sometimes because they did not come a month sooner. Did they come too soon or too late? They may be frustrated if satisfactory answers are not available. How is a patient to know when, or if, to come?

Medical care for back pain should be sought if any of the following conditions is present:

1. Back pain follows an impact injury or accident, as stated earlier in this book.

2. Back pain gets worse, not better, after a couple of days of rest, or if it continues for two, three, or more weeks.

3. Back pain interferes with sleep.

4. Back pain is accompanied by fever or urinary problems. Difficulty in urinating is an emergency and is one of the few reasons for urgent surgery, perhaps to free a nerve root that has become entrapped by pressure of disc or bone.

5. Back pain is accompanied by feelings of tingling, numbness, or weakness in the lower limbs. There could be pressure on a nerve that may need to be corrected surgically.

6. There is sciatic pain down the back of the leg, especially if it is felt below the level of the knee.

7. There is swelling or pain in other joints, or pain in any other part of the body.

8. There is unexplained weight loss.

9. Self-help efforts are just not working and there is a sense that a doctor is needed.

WHERE TO GO FIRST, AND THEN WHAT?

First see someone you have seen before and with whom you have at least some acquaintance, even if it is clear that this person is not a back expert. The person may be a family physician, a specialist in internal medicine, or a nurse practitioner. Conceivably, he or she could even be a specialist in a field far removed from back care but with whom you have an ongoing relationship. This person could certainly expedite a responsible referral to a medical colleague.

If you are a member of a health maintenance organization (HMO), you must choose your provider from those within the organization, or you can choose to pay for the "outside" consultation yourself. You may wish to do this. On the other hand, the organization may provide a referral network so that you do not have to do an extensive outside search for specialists. If the outside referral is made by the HMO, it should be paid for by the HMO. It is important to understand your health insurance and to be comfortable with your choice. Most employers offer several health insurance options as required by law. The coverage and requirements can be explained by your benefits or personnel office, or by that of the employed family member through whom you have coverage as a spouse or child. Get up-to-date descriptive booklets and read them.

The temptation may be to go to the hospital emergency room, but this may not be the best decision. Although a doctor may be seen at the hospital within an hour or two, instead of a day or two, or even as much as a week or more, the hospital emergency room in teaching hospitals will be staffed by physicians in training, not spine specialists, such as orthopedists or neurosurgeons, even though house staff have access to specialists. The house staff will decide whether to admit the patient to the hospital.

Communication between physician and patient is always important, especially in certain areas of health and medicine, and back care is one of them. Back pain can be elusive, intermittent, and described only in vague terms. Often a diagnosis is hard to pinpoint. Even when one can, what to do can be problematic. And different specialties frequently have different solutions for the same back problem.

The patient's tasks include learning as much as possible about the problem and about the available medical resources. The patient must then describe the relevant symptoms as accurately, concisely, and completely as possible and answer physician questions in the same manner. The patient must then be prepared to ask questions that will elicit desired information.

Bringing another person along for the discussion portion of the visit is usually a major help in obtaining as much information as possible, acting to prevent the patient from feeling overwhelmed by the medical environment and the "expert" to the extent that essential questions often remain unasked. Seeing the physician as an authority figure instead of a knowledgeable consultant inhibits the patient's ability to obtain important information.

Keep in mind the likelihood, even the certainty, of the need for a second opinion, and possibly a third, fourth, or fifth, even if the insurance coverage requires a second opinion only. The physician may make a referral, either immediately or after another visit or two. Or the patient may decide to see someone else. The purpose may be to obtain another opinion, get more information, or select another physician who appears more appropriate.

Changing physicians in "midstream" does not require "going back to square one" in medical care. When seeing patients, physicians depend on records and lab results, not on whether the patient has previously been in the office, and records can be transferred from the previous physician's office. In most states you can obtain copies of your own medical records from hospitals or clinics. You can then maintain your own files for your information and for medical care you may need in the future. Physicians' office records may not be available, but physicians will prepare notes summarizing their findings for the use of other physicians.

Because back surgery does not have the predictable outcome of many of the more standard surgeries, back patients, like cancer patients, or others with certain medical conditions, may often be well served by contacting out-of-area facilities in addition to local medical resources. Note also that back surgery can be done by two separate medical specialists, orthopedic surgeons and neurosurgeons.

Some spine specialists will see patients only on a referral basis, requiring that patients be referred by another physician. Knowing the medical system and being able to insert oneself into it may bring better access to those physicians who feel the need to limit their accessibility to the public at large. They may or may not be better doctors, but they are either very busy or limiting the nature of their work they choose to do. One source that may be useful in selecting a physician is the hospital nursing administration.

The decision to have a disc partially or wholly removed, spinal bones cut into, or spinal nerves manipulated is a major consideration. Equally, it is a major decision to do nothing when the patient is experiencing serious pain and disability. Braces, traction, body casts, and chiropractic treatments are not to be accepted lightly either, even though all may have a place in resolving specific medical problems. On the other hand, when the patient is partly or wholly disabled, in chronic pain and overwhelmed by feelings of powerlessness and ignorance, it is easy to understand many patients' desperate pleas to "do something, Doctor. Do anything."

Before any procedure is considered, unless there is difficulty with urination, which is an obvious emergency, as accurate a diagnosis as possible is needed. This is primary, even knowing the difficulties in obtaining it and the interrelationship of the structures of the back. The first step in diagnosis is a complete medical history. This may be followed by selected medical tests.

Then, before any procedure is undertaken, the patient needs to know how frequently it is performed: in the country as a whole, at the selected hospital, and by the physician who recommends it or is planning to do it. What are the expected benefits, and what are the possible risks? What have been the long-term results? Can the surgery or procedure make the problem worse? What are the statistics? What exactly is the procedure, step by step? Is it useful to speak ahead of time with the anesthesiologist? Is it possible to talk, with their permission, to former patients who have had the procedure? What is involved in recovery? Is informational literature available that could be useful to you? What articles have been written on the procedure?

It must be recognized that many studies are preliminary or inconclusive. And, as will be discussed later in the chapter, there are inherent difficulties in accurate assessments of the patient's outcome. An analysis of the patient's pain is largely dependent on the patient's reports. Even evaluation of range of motion has a subjective element that is difficult to avoid. There are other obstacles in the way of obtaining accurate evaluations. Furthermore, what information there is has not been generally accessible to the public.

As indicated at the beginning of this book, back care involves a number of professional disciplines. Before providing an overview of possible medical tests that may lead to that all-important diagnosis, a summary of the spheres of interest of these disciplines is offered. The professional organizations of each can provide additional information.

INTRODUCING THE BACK SPECIALISTS

The *orthopedist* or *orthopedic surgeon* is a physician who has had several additional years of training beyond medical school. This person may be board-certified, meaning that the specialty exams have been passed, or may be board-qualified, meaning that he or she is eligible to take the exams but has not yet taken or passed them.

The orthopedist diagnoses and treats, with surgical or nonsurgical methods, bone, muscle, and joint disorders. This specialty is concerned with preservation and restoration of the skeletal system, joints, and associated structures.

The *neurologist* is a physician with several additional years of training beyond medical school, who may be board-certified or board-qualified, and who is expert in the diagnosis and nonsurgical treatment of conditions of the neuromuscular system, spinal cord, and nervous system.

The *neurosurgeon* is a physician, again with several

additional years of training in a hospital residency program. Whether the physician is board-certified, or board-qualified and not yet board-certified may not relate directly to the degree of competency, as with other specialties.

The neurosurgeon performs surgery on the nervous system and treats back problems with surgery. If the problem appears to be one of sciatic pain, nerve entrapment, or primarily a nerve problem, many suggest consultation with a neurosurgeon.

Spinal fusion surgery involving bone grafts is done by orthopedic surgeons. The common back surgeries can, however, be done either by a neurosurgeon or an orthopedic surgeon. Their particular interests, training, and experience may be the deciding factors in selecting a surgeon. Still, knowledgeable medical professionals express the opinion that bone and joint back surgery and scoliosis treatment should be done by orthopedists and that neurosurgeons should do surgical procedures involving discs and all surgery involving freeing nerves entrapped by encroachment of bone or disc.

An *internist* is a physician, again board-qualified or board-certified, who specializes in the diagnosis and medical, nonsurgical treatment of diseases of adults with the exception of obstetrical problems. The internist may be the initial caregiver for gynecological problems. This *specialist in internal medicine* is not to be confused with the medical intern, who has a year of additional training after receiving the M.D. degree.

The internist may diagnose tumors in the spine or other parts of the body, and diagnose and treat arthritis or other systemic illnesses or conditions that may have back pain as a symptom. When a number of specialists are involved in a problem the internist may be seen as a coordinator of the patient's care. However, because there are often practical obstacles to achieving this goal, the patient should not abdicate his or her own coordinating role.

The *radiologist* is a physician with four years or more of graduate training in radiology. As with other medical specialists, the radiologist may be board-qualified or board-certified. The radiologist's role in diagnosing medical problems, including back problems, has burgeoned during recent years with the explosion of new imaging technology impacting on diagnostic testing. Ultrasound and other, more recent technologies are available for better visualization of many body structures. Radiologic expertise is required to perform many of the diagnostic procedures and, of course, to evaluate the subsequent results.

Because accurate diagnosis of a back problem is a prerequisite to considering or pursuing any of the myriad forms of medical treatment, the role of the radiologist is pivotal.

The *neuroradiologist* is a radiologist with special expertise in diagnosing nerve problems that can be seen on film. Neuroradiology is a subspecialty of radiology.

The patient ordinarily has limited access to the radiologist, who is hired by the hospital or medical group. Radiologic findings are communicated directly to the patient's physician.

The *osteopath* has an D.O. degree instead of an M.D. degree and therefore is not a medical doctor. Osteopaths may use manipulation therapy or other hands-on therapy in the diagnosis and treatment of back problems.

Osteopathy is a system of therapy founded by Andrew Taylor (1828–1917) and is based on the theory of the body's capacity to make its own remedies against disease when it is in a normal structural relationship in favorable environmental conditions and with adequate nutrition. Osteopaths accept physical, medicinal, and surgical methods of diagnosis and therapy while placing chief emphasis on the importance of normal body mechanics and manipulative methods of detecting and correcting faulty structure.

The *physiatrist,* a lesser-known specialist to most,

might be found in a pain center or medical rehabilitation center. The physiatrist, not a physical therapist, is a physician who specializes in physical medicine and rehabilitation to treat muscle and bone disorders. Therapies include exercises, heat, traction, cold therapy, and electrical stimulation of muscles.

Chiropractors are not medical doctors. They have a doctoral degree in their field and are addressed as doctors. They may use manipulation, heat, acupuncture, ultrasound, massage, or hydrotherapy. They may prescribe exercises. For decades controversies have swirled around chiropractors, partly reflecting the complexities and uncertainties of back pain. Controversy continues. Many loyal patients have sworn to the effectiveness of their chiropractic help in relieving back muscle spasm even as physicians have found it difficult to document the success and stated that manipulation can make some back problems worse. Physicians have feared, too, that chiropractors may become involved in problems beyond their expertise and that chiropractors, at least in the past, have attributed far too many human ills to spinal misalignment.

As medical insurance begins to cover some chiropractic treatment, chiropractors are being seen in selected cases as having useful services to perform, and occasionally they may even receive physician referrals. All fifty states now license and officially recognize chiropractics as a health profession. Medicare, Medicaid, and Workers' Compensation honor the insurance claims for chiropractic treatment. Chiropractors treat back, neck, and other musculoskeletal ailments, and their patients number more than ten million.

Chiropractors cannot prescribe medication or perform surgery. They often see patients for a series of treatments. Spinal X rays are used as a diagnostic tool, and many chiropractors require a substantial number of X-ray films. Patients may discuss the necessity and the consequent X-ray exposure with the practitioner and with other specialists knowledgeable about X-ray exposure.

Chiropractors use a system of therapeutics based on the claim that disease is caused by abnormal function of the nervous system. The attempt is made to restore normal function of the nervous system by manipulation and treatment of structures of the human body, especially those of the spinal column.

The physical exam includes postural studies, range of motion, and palpation of the spine for tenderness or bumps. Treatment involves correcting a diagnosed misalignment, whether or not it can be shown on X-ray, and restoring mobility. This may include a rapid downward pressure thrust on the spine, which may result in an audible, although usually painless, click.

Chiropractors have four years of graduate classroom and clinical training, including all medical school subjects except surgery and pharmacology. Graduates must pass an exam of the National Board of Chiropractic Examiners to be eligible for state licensing.

Physical therapists are graduates of a school of physical therapy and receive a P.T. degree. Insurance coverage and medical policy may require that patients be referred by a physician. Contact between physician and therapist is maintained, and written notes are inserted into the medical record of the hospital or group practice if this is the setting for medical care.

Patients may be referred early in the assessment of back pain or as part of the rehabilitative process after an accident or surgery. The patient may be seen once or many times.

Physical therapists assess muscular strength and flexibility issues and may demonstrate to the patient the prescribed exercises to be done on a regular basis at home. Physical therapists assist in rehabilitation and restoration of normal bodily function after illness or injury and may use massage, manipulation, hydrotherapy, or various forms of energy such as electric or ultrasound.

Family physicians do an initial assessment, order tests, give advice on back care, and assist with referrals to specialists when and if needed.

Nursing staff members may do preliminary assessment and offer life-style suggestions. They assist with referrals to physicians.

TAKING THE TESTS

There are issues both in taking diagnostic tests and in grading these tests. Doing some homework ahead of time can be worthwhile in reassuring the patient.

One or more "positive" tests does not necessarily mean that surgery will be required. Surgery does not always help, and it can sometimes make the patient feel worse. Problems that appear severe may resolve themselves in that the pain does eventually lessen. In fact, most back surgery is described as "elective."

As explained earlier, backs can have one or many structural abnormalities and still present no pain. Even obvious deformities may not be painful. Or there *is* pain, and the tests come back negative, indicating that there is no problem. Back specialists have noted that a disc may be shown to be bulging. But even after surgery there might still be pain originating in another location, perhaps another disc. The problem could even be in the hip, and not in the back at all. Therefore, it is no surprise to find that more than one test may be required.

Medical practitioners often have their favorite tests in which they have confidence in accordance with their experience, training, and the facilities available at their institution. Not all tests are available at every medical center. Some are simple office tests. Others involve dyes and radiation and are known as "invasive" tests. "Noninvasive" tests include office tests and technology such as ultrasound (not usually part of back workups) and other imaging techniques requiring neither radiation exposure nor the use of substances that penetrate the body. This book will give you an overview by summarizing the possible diagnostic procedures.

Office Tests

These usually consist of a simple range of motion tests. While standing, how far can the patient bend forward? To the side? Backward? Patients often have some trepidation while complying with directions to bend, fearing that these motions may increase the extent of the injury or make the pain worse, even if only temporarily. But the physician needs documentation of the problem both for the preliminary assessment and as a comparison for the future.

The patient may be asked to stand up on the toes and on back on the heels to ascertain possible pressure on nerves. Is there pain in the legs and, if so, where and to what extent? Are there areas of numbness? Is the circumference of one leg markedly less than that of the other, indicating possible pressure on nerves, with consequent reduced muscle activity and, therefore, muscle size because muscle fibers are stimulated by nerves? Knee and ankle reflexes may be checked, also to assess nerve function.

The straight leg raise test may be done to check for a possible disc problem. The patient raises the straightened leg perpendicular to the body, or the physician raises the leg to this position. If this is impossible or results in severe pain, there is a possibility of a herniated or ruptured disc.

A blood test may be done to help rule out inflammatory processes such as certain forms of arthritis or other medical conditions.

Most backaches improve within a few weeks, but at the next visit, perhaps several weeks later or less, the physician and patient may decide that they need more information. Hospital diagnostic procedures may be indicated as the next logical step. Again, even positive tests do not mean that the physician will suggest immediate or future surgery.

Hospital Diagnostic Procedures

Before considering or undergoing hospital tests, many people have almost no understanding of what to expect, what will be done, or even what might be learned. They have doubts and fears, but in the stress of their office visits they are unsure what questions need to be asked and answered. How articulate can they be in a territory that is largely unknown to the public? Back care is a field in which the experts do not always agree and about which there is still much to learn.

Some physicians have a skeleton or model spine in their offices. If so, patients should have the possible problem and the prospective test described, with the skeletal model used for purposes of demonstration. Models, photos, and sample diagnostic X rays are useful, too, but lack the third dimension, which helps immeasurably in putting back structures into perspective. Textbook illustrations can be used to illustrate the back and the nervous system, including the downward sweep from the spinal cord of nerves exiting from the cord's lower portion. These are often described as the "horse's tail."

The following questions are suggested as guides for each test under consideration. Knowing the questions ahead of time can make office visits more useful and meet the needs of both physician and patient more efficiently. Of course, additional visits or phone calls may also occur, but knowing as much as possible ahead of time tends to circumvent possible confusion or dissatisfaction later.

1. How reliable are the test results? What is the percentage of test results that will show a problem when there is not one, and how many will show that there is not a problem when there actually is one? (This is also known as percentage of "false positive" and "false negative.")

2. How will the test results, whether positive or negative, alter any proposed treatment or procedure? If it is clear that surgery at this time would be premature and the test involves certain risks or discomforts, is there a reason to do the test now?

3. What information can the test be expected to give? What might it reveal in regard to problems with the vertebrae, discs, muscles, or nerves?

4. What, if any, are the risks involved in the test, and how likely are they to occur? What pain should you expect during the procedure and afterward?

5. What is the sequence of events? Where is the test done, and how is it scheduled? What is the anticipated length of the test? Who does the procedure? Exactly what happens during the test?

6. When will the test results be available? Should the patient call the physician's office for them, or will the physician's office notify the patient? Will an office visit be scheduled at that time?

It is likely that a series of *spinal X rays* will be the first test ordered. X rays will be taken from several angles to obtain as complete information on the general configuration of the spine as possible. A substantial dose of radiation is received by the patient (if the patient is pregnant the X ray should not be done). Men should request a lead shield to protect the testes. Women, on the other hand, cannot protect the reproductive organs and genetic material because a lead shield over the ovaries would cover up the lumbar-sacral area; for any other part of the back a lead shield should be used.

Even though X-ray results are not used as the sole basis for determining a need for surgery, a lot can be learned from them. X rays show bones but not discs. Disc spaces between the vertebrae revealed in X rays are significant. However, as previously described, the disc space does not tend to narrow immediately even when a disc ruptures.

X rays also show the alignment of the spinal bones. The picture is two-dimensional, but the oblique views from another angle help to piece the information together. Scoliosis, the sideways bending of the spinal column previously described, can be seen, as can evidence of osteoporosis. Infections of the bone may be observed along with any destruction of bone by tumor. Sacralization, formation of an extra joint resulting from the joining of the winged projections of a vertebra to its neighbor on one side and that can contribute to rotational stress on the spine, especially if in daily life proper body mechanics are not maintained, can also be seen in X rays. Vertebral fractures may appear on X-ray film, although some are hard to see.

Osteophytes are commonly observed on X rays. These extra bony growths on vertebrae are especially problematic in mid life and later and result from the pressure of bone on bone as disc spaces narrow with age. Wear and tear on facet joints resulting from repeated heavy lifting or excessive back arching may show up on an X ray and, along with disc height loss, contribute to the growth of those frequently seen osteophytes.

With advancing age spinal X rays are likely to show narrowed disc spaces indicating the "normal" disc degeneration, evidence of osteoporosis, and the presence of osteophytes. Occupational health studies have shown X-ray changes correlating with heavy lifting in the workplace by laborers, but there is yet no way of knowing just how these anticipated, "normal" changes in the back can be slowed by proper back care throughout life.

Electromyography offers the opportunity to study and record the electrical conduction patterns of skeletal muscle. In Greek the word *myelo* means muscle. Needle electrodes are inserted into muscle. The test helps to identify abnormal muscular activity in muscles supplied by the sciatic nerve, helping to identify a possible disc problem. No radiation is involved.

For a *Discogram* a needle is inserted through the lower back into the suspected disc, a dye is injected, and an X ray is taken. An abnormal disc may be detected by the pattern of absorption of the dye. An abnormal disc absorbs more of the injection substance. However, interpretation of this test can be difficult, and radiation exposure is involved. Discograms are done rarely, if ever.

A *myelogram* requires a dye to be inserted by needle into the space around the spinal cord. Then, when X-ray films are taken, an obstruction or abnormal configuration may be seen on the film. The radiologist may spot an abnormal disc or even a tumor. It is possible to miss a disc problem with a myelogram, and they are done only if spinal surgery is proposed, not during the early weeks of back pain.

The myelogram has the following risks:

1. Nausea and vomiting are common, but they disappear usually within a few hours to one day.

2. Spinal headaches may occur due to leakage of cerebrospinal fluid through the puncture site. It usually resolves spontaneously within a few days. The spinal headache goes away if the patient lies fairly flat but gets worse if the patient sits or stands.

3. Seizures are related to the dye getting into the ventricles, or spaces, in the brain. This is uncommon but is a risk. The seizures are transient and go away when the dye is cleared out of the system. This complication is more common in cervical myelograms of the neck region but is rare in lumbar myelograms. Radiologists are very careful not to let the dye go into the head.

   The risk of seizures is increased if the patient has had previous seizures, is on antipsychotic drugs, or is on some of the antinausea drugs such as Compazine.

4. A possible delayed complication is pain caused by inflammation of the spinal nerves and arachnoiditis (inflammation of a membrane in the brain). With newer dyes these problems have become uncommon.

5. Very rarely, if the study is not done in a sterile fashion, an infection, such as meningitis, may occur.

Myelograms, although relatively inexpensive, are now being replaced by more recent technology.

Bone scans may be used to diagnose fractures, tumors, or arthritis. The scan is a two-dimensional image of the gamma rays emitted by a radioisotope, revealing the varying concentration of a specific body tissue. Brain, thyroid, and other types of scans are also done. Radiation exposure is involved but is less than for most X-ray exams.

The *CT scan,* formerly known as the *CAT scan,* is frequently done before considering a myelogram. Most medical centers have this capability. Some share the equipment with a neighboring hospital.

CT is an abbreviation of the term "computerized tomography." A tomograph is an X-ray apparatus that images a layer of tissue at any depth. The CT scan utilizes an X-ray machine that rotates around the body to produce horizontal X-ray "slices." The computer then transforms the information into film that can be read by a radiologist. CT is a sophisticated form of imaging. A herniated disc or a narrowed spinal canal due to encroaching bone may be diagnosed using a CT scan. However, despite the clear images produced, the CT scan can miss a disc problem.

The CT scan can identify herniated discs in the lumbar spine but not in the neck (cervical spine) and chest (thoracic portion of the spine). For these a myelogram is done prior to the CT scan. The CT scan in cervical and thoracic regions is useful for bony problems, but myelographic dye needs to be put into the space at the top part of the spinal cord near the brain membranes (called the subarachnoid space) before a disc herniation or bulge can be seen.

Magnetic resonance imaging, called *MRI,* is a remarkable, complex new diagnostic technology. With MRI, nerves, spinal cord, discs, spinal cysts, and tumors can all be clearly seen. It shows inflammation and fluid buildup and can even see into bone marrow. MRI is an excellent diagnostic tool for back problems and for many other medical problems as well. It is the very latest in radiologic technology and may supplant the myelogram. MRI was first used diagnostically in 1973, and since then its medical implications have been explored rapidly.

MRI involves neither radiation exposure for the patient nor the injection of dye. Not yet universally available, it operates using the principles of magnetism and high-frequency radio waves. Radio waves are part of the electromagnetic spectrum, which includes visible light and X rays. MRI is not to be confused with *ultrasound,* not usually part of a back pain workup. Ultrasound is based on the use of low-frequency sound waves, related to pressure waves transmitted through air, water, or solids, which are bounced off tissues and, like MRI, involve no radiation exposure. Ultrasound uses the same principles as *sonar.*

The patient is positioned on a table in a large, tube-shaped magnet. The powerful magnetic field results in temporary changes in the atoms of the body. The body contains many hydrogen atoms, each containing an electron and a proton. With magnetization, the protons line up in a certain pattern. With application of oscillating high-frequency sound waves, energy is absorbed and released. The time required for the protons in various body tissue to return to their original status after magnetization is measured.

A major advantage of MRI over CT is that body tissues are visualized in any slice or orientation desired. Having an MRI is similar to having a CT scan, except that MRI scans are very noisy, with "tapping" sounds during the time that radio wave pulses are directed at the patient, although the sounds are not from the radio waves but originate within the equipment.

MORE ON DIAGNOSIS

What else is being diagnosed with these diagnostic tests and the resulting films? Many of the possible medical conditions have been addressed earlier in the context of informing you how your back is put together, how you can take care of it, and explaining the possible benefits of diagnostic tests.

Disc problems have been described, along with possible facet joint problems, osteoporosis, and scoliosis. Additional comments will be offered on the latter three conditions and on several other back problems.

A more complete overview and orientation are offered here for better understanding of what can happen to the back. If you do have a medical problem, knowing the details may help you to feel more competent in obtaining professional help.

FACET JOINTS AND ARTHRITIC CHANGES

As disc spaces shrink and the vertebrae are brought closer together, the likelihood of wear and tear, osteophyte formation, and bone spurs on the vertebrae may be increased. Osteoarthritis or degenerative arthritis of the spine, which may be present, is an inflammatory process resulting from bone rubbing against bone, causing bony growths and irritation. Subluxation, or partial dislocation, of facet joints may occur as disc spaces diminish in height and vertebral changes occur, especially in the bony projections on the sides and back of each vertebra. The result may be a poorer "fit" of the joints during back flexion, back extension, and lateral bending.

In tribal societies back pain and disc degeneration are minimal, both clinically and radiologically. This means that in these societies there are few back pain complaints and that X rays do not show the expected degenerative changes. The "whys" have not been studied.

Osteoarthritis affects more than one region of the spine and is especially prevalent among the older population and among manual laborers. There may or may not be symptoms.

Rheumatoid arthritis, often a disease of the younger population and most common in women, affects other parts of the body, such as the hands, more often than it does the spine. It is a systemic disease resulting in joint inflammation. Its cause is unknown.

OSTEOPOROSIS

Bone demineralization and degeneration result in increasing difficulty in supporting the upper part of the body. The lower thoracic and lumbar regions tend to compress together to form a rounded back; this is osteoporosis.

Nerve entrapment can occur in osteoporosis and also in osteoarthritis as bony configurations change.

SPINAL STENOSIS

Another bone problem, stenosis, occurs when the spinal canal narrows due to encroachment of bone, resulting in inadequate space for nerves. The condition can be congenital, but it can result from wear and tear changes. Bony growths and bone spurs impinge on the hollow space in each vertebral bone. This most often occurs in people over fifty.

Stenosis may be a result of the previous loss of a disc, perhaps because of disc surgery. Then, with the passage of time, increased spinal pressures may encourage bony overgrowth that narrows the spinal canal.

SCOLIOSIS

The sideways bending of the spine, to a slight degree, is not uncommon among the population at large. However, the curvature can become pronounced and obvious, and aggressive treatment is required to prevent its continued progression. Severe scoliosis can interfere with the expansion of the lungs.

One can be born with scoliosis or develop it later. It is often described as a condition occurring most frequently in teenage girls. The reasons are unclear and the cause may be missing muscles, weak muscles on one side of the back, a short leg, a deformed vertebra, or severe back muscle spasm. If the back is already sinking to one side, it will tend to continue to sink under stresses of gravity.

SPONDYLITIS

Spondylitis is a Greek-derived word meaning inflammation of the vertebrae. *Ankylosing spondylitis* means stiffening of the spine. It is an arthritic disease, and the back becomes rigid and gradually fuses to bone. There may be difficulty in expanding the chest as the body bends forward. Breathing becomes difficult. The spine and sacroiliac joints are affected. It is a disease with a strong hereditary component and is most common in men. It is much less common than the rheumatoid arthritis described earlier.

No prevention is known, but exercises, a possible brace, or even surgical straightening of the spine may be considered.

SPONDYLOLISTHESIS

Spondylolisthesis literally means "slipping vertebrae." It is a forward displacement of one vertebra over another one. The lowest lumbar vertebra slips over the sacrum or the fourth lumbar vertebra slips over the fifth or lowest lumbar vertebra, the location of the arch of the back. This may also affect the alignment of the several vertebrae above the slippage. A brace or possible spinal fusion surgery may be prescribed. Usually it is impossible to put the vertebra back into its original spot, but further slippage can be prevented. For the degenerative form of slippage spinal nerves may become entrapped and have to be freed. In younger people this condition involves a fracture through the spine.

The cause can be congenital, as a consequence of variations in the formation of the lower spine above the sacrum. It can result from severe mechanical injury.

Spondylolysis is a similar word, but it refers to flattening or dissolution of bony parts of the spine. The cause can be congenital.

OSTEOMYELITIS

Osteomyelitis is an infection in the bone, most often due to skin bacteria. Bacteria enter the body, perhaps through a cut, and are carried around the body by the bloodstream. If resistance is low, it is possible for an infection to develop at a site within the body, including the spine.

BONE FRACTURES

Bones may break or crack through injury or when weakened by osteoporosis. No special treatment may be indicated or possible even if the fracture shows up on X ray. Hips may also break due to the processes of osteoporosis.

SYSTEMIC ILLNESS AND BACK PAIN

Back pain can be a signal that there is illness elsewhere in the body but not originating in the back itself. Problems of the kidneys, intestines, pancreas, uterus, ovaries, or prostate gland can result in back pain. Vascular diseases, hip problems, and even ulcers can be associated with back pain. The importance of a complete physical exam and the receipt of an accurate diagnosis before undertaking any course of treatment are underscored by considering that the source of back pain may not even be primarily the back.

"TAKING THE CURE"

Back treatments are wide-ranging, all the way from aspirin to back braces, acupuncture, hormones, and major surgery. Knowing the fundamentals of possible back problems is useful in understanding why there are so many approaches to treatment.

First, there are the nonsurgical treatments, designated the conservative treatments with the possible exception of chiropractics, depending on personal and professional factors. Because back pain episodes often resolve themselves within a few weeks, sometimes returning later, evaluating methods of treatment is not as easy as might at first appear. Physicians, therefore, within certain parameters, may leave decisions to the patient. "Try it. See if it helps."

REST

Rest has been discussed extensively in this book. The principle is to allow inflammatory processes to recede and for the patient and physician to gain better understanding of the cause of the pain. At the same time, necessary rest must be balanced with the need to maintain muscle tone and avoid bone demineralization.

WEIGHT LOSS

If there is obvious excess body weight, the need for loss of these extra pounds must be addressed.

ASPIRIN

The physician may suggest aspirin for pain relief and as an anti-inflammatory agent. Other pain killing medication may be suggested.

TRANQUILIZERS

These are less likely these days to be prescribed by the physician. The purpose of tranquilizers is to reduce mus-

cle tension. However, they may have addictive properties, and the problem of muscle tension can also be at-
tacked in other ways, such as learning and practicing
relaxation techniques, use of heat, massage, and biofeedback.

BIOFEEDBACK

Visual or auditory feedback is given as the patient relaxes
or tenses. The feedback may reflect increased muscle
tension, increased heart rate, hand warmth reflecting the
amount of blood flow, or evidence of physiological
change. It has been used to teach groups of patients to
relax their back muscles and reduce back pain.

MASSAGE

Massage may be used to reduce stress and aid muscular
relaxation. It can increase blood supply to muscles and
has other physiological benefits as well, including relief
of muscle spasm. Spinal manipulation therapy has been
reported to have the same benefits.

ACUPUNCTURE

The insertion of needles at specific body locations can
alleviate pain transmitted by nerve pathways. Exactly
how it works is not known, but trained practitioners have
used it for centuries to relieve pain resulting from many
causes. *Acupressure* uses pressure points on the body to
alter body function and relieve pain.

TRACTION

While many of the above therapies work on the principles of decreasing muscle spasm and increasing muscle relaxation, traction does not. Most of the above therapies are not focused directly on relieving disc or spinal alignment problems.

Traction is not a frequently used method of treatment, and there are a number of unanswered questions about the process. But it has appeared to help some people and it has a plausible rationale, even though for some it can increase their pain. By separating vertebrae and enlarging disc spaces the spinal alignment may be corrected. Traction can be used for necks as well as backs. The "placebo effect" can make it difficult to evaluate because it is known that the patient can feel better just because a treatment is being administered. Many physicians feel that the benefits of traction may be short-lived.

In traction weights are used to increase the separation between the vertebrae. The number of pounds used and the period of time the force is maintained vary greatly, depending on the orthopedist. All agree that it must be used with caution. There is no evidence that it permanently changes spinal alignment or that it allows a protruding disc to reposition itself, although the possibility exists that the changed mechanical forces might affect the disc.

THE "HANGING" THERAPIES

Several years ago equipment was developed to allow people to hang upside down with their feet encased in boots. Prior to that, people, especially those with a curve, as in scoliosis, hung from horizontal bars or even tree branches to help straighten spines. Hanging acts to stretch muscles that may be tight on one side of the back. "Hanging" therapy is similar to traction, but the weight is that of the patient's own body instead of having two opposing forces, one pulling on the lower half of the body and the other pulling the upper part of the body in the opposite direction.

The "hanging" therapy has been shown to increase blood pressure readings, and there have been other sources of apprehension, including effects on ankles and knees. It is suggested that instead one suspend the body from the thighs or have a tilt table for which the angle of incline can be selected.

BRACES, CORSETS, AND CASTS

Only an orthopedist can recommend the proper type of brace, corset, or cast to be used. Sometimes they are used after surgery to restrict certain motions during the period of healing. They may increase comfort at times for some. However, they can permit abdominal muscles to weaken if overused or used inappropriately, and by immobilizing one part of the spine, the forces on another part may be increased. The correct design for the desired use is all-important. The correction of deforming scoliosis is an important use of these devices.

EXERCISE

Again, exercise is of major importance in the treatment and prevention of back problems. Essentially, back fitness is what this book is all about.

The treatment of osteoporosis includes back extension exercises to help prevent further bone loss. It includes dietary advice as well, and for postmenopausal women there may also be discussion of the use of estrogen. Many, including women's health consumer groups, express doubts about both the need and the possible long-term carcinogenic effects of prescribing estrogen on a mass basis for this purpose, recommending instead a program of adequate weight-bearing exercise and a diet rich in calcium and other minerals.

"UNDER THE KNIFE"

Actually, not all back surgery involves use of the surgical knife. One procedure involves dissolving tissue chemically. This section will acquaint you with the benefits and, at times, lack of benefit or even possible risks of the common surgical interventions.

"My cousin had his spine fused." "My doctor is thinking about doing an operation on my disc." "I hear that back surgery is risky." "What does all this mean?" "What are the success rates?" These are all very common questions about back surgery.

Taking the last question first, the success rates are stated as being from 70 to 90 percent, no matter what form of treatment—surgical or not—is selected. Most patients tend to get better, even those with sciatica or other evidence of disc problems. When two groups of patients are compared after a period of months, or longer, one who had surgery and one who did not, there may be little difference in the pain reported by the two groups. But when questioned soon after the surgery, those with surgery reported less pain than the other group. Some patients have had two or three surgeries, including a repeat of a procedure, and still report back pain.

It is difficult to match the two groups. The time frame used affects results, whether patients are questioned at two months or five years. Long-term follow-up is difficult. Samples may be small. Reports are subjective. The researcher must depend on patient reports. Did the patient have the pain for months or years, or for six to eight weeks before having surgery? The surgical outcome appears to be better if the pain is of more recent origin—for example, a couple of months. At the same time, surgery must not be done without adequate diagnosis and without allowing time for the body's own healing mechanisms to work. Also, the procedure may have minor variations, depending on what the surgeon finds. Patients who work on their problem by exercising, losing weight, and bending and lifting properly can be expected to show better results. The patient's attention to self-care, or lack of it, may not be taken into account when subsequently assessing the results of surgery.

The success rate of a surgical procedure depends a great deal on how carefully the patients are selected; the patient's attitude toward the procedure is also a factor. As previously said, most back surgery is considered to be elective. The procedure must be the one that can help the particular problem the patient has. For carefully selected patients an operation can be exactly what that patient needs.

CHYMOPAPAIN

Chymopapain is an enzyme that acts to dissolve tissue. It is an enzyme derived from papaya leaves and is used in meat tenderizer. First used in experimental tests in Chicago, it was in fairly extensive use in certain medical centers by the early 1970s. Later it received U.S. Food and Drug Administration approval. Lately the procedure has fallen out of favor.

The enzyme dissolves disc material, but not nerves unless injected directly into them.

Good results have been obtained using chymopapain, about the same as with other medical or surgical treatments. Disc pressure on nerves is usually relieved. However, in some cases the patient might be allergic to the chymopapain (one of every five hundred), and the reaction could be fatal. About half of all patients have severe back pain for several weeks following the injection, probably due to inflammation of the nerves. The loss of disc height after the dissolution of the disc is thought by some doctors to cause increased osteoarthritic changes in the spine in later life.

DISKECTOMY OR DISC EXCISION

The surgeon goes in from the back to remove free fragments or portions of the disc. The entire disc is usually not removed. The purpose is to relieve the pressure of a protruding disc or a disc fragment on a nerve root.

The first disc operation was performed in Boston in 1934 by a team comprised of an orthopedic surgeon and a neurosurgeon who removed the disc and then fused the two vertebrae above and below the disc. However, disc material can be removed without fusing the vertebrae. Fusions have become less frequent in recent years and will be discussed in a separate section.

Most disc surgery involves removing displaced disc material. Some vertebral bone is removed to gain access to the disc, and perhaps some of the ligament. The nerves are also moved aside to gain access to the disc. In addition, the surgeon will free nerve roots from scar tissue and make sure that no structure is compressing them. Sometimes the scar tissue is from previous back surgery. Repeat surgery also carries with it the risk of producing scar tissue. Disc fragments may be removed or the inner soft part of the disc, but the fibrous outer portion of the disc usually remains.

Although the spine may be somewhat less stable after surgery, depending on how much material was removed, this is noticeable only when unusual stress is placed on the back. There may also be some change in the spine mechanics, which the patient may or may not notice.

More recently a less traumatic microsurgical procedure has been introduced to remove disc fragments. Another new surgical procedure, designed for unfragmented herniated discs and performed under local anesthesia, involves inserting a specially designed needle with a rotary blade into the disc, grinding the disc material, and suctioning it back through the needle.

LAMINECTOMY

The removal of disc material involves going through part of the bony spinal ring to expose the bulging disc. The lamina, a thin part of the vertebra, can be removed without compromising the stability of the spine to any significant degree.

In spinal stenosis, in which there is bony overgrowth resulting in narrowing the spinal canal, bone may have to be removed to relieve pressure on nerve roots. Other bony growths may be removed, as on facet joints.

SPINAL FUSION

Formerly, spinal fusion was done more often than it is now, but there are certain conditions under which it may be used to restore stability to the spine. Its purpose is to form a connection between or among two or more vertebrae.

Bone from the patient's body, most often from the pelvis, is grafted onto the living bone of the spine. Several months may be required for the graft to "take." Grafts are gradually replaced by the patient's own bone. If the graft does not "take," the fusion must be repeated.

Most fusions are posterior fusions, meaning that the surgeon enters from the direction of the patient's back to approach the vertebrae for surgery. The grafts are vertical. Rarely, an anterior interbody fusion is done in which the disc is replaced by a bone graft. The surgeon places the bone graft in the space previously occupied by the disc instead of fusing the vertebrae by connecting posterior vertebral bones with the vertical grafts. The latter surgery has more risks.

At times when a diskectomy has not helped, the surgeon performs a fusion as the second surgery. This is not usual, except perhaps for a patient who must perform heavy lifting as a condition of employment. A fusion may be done for spondylolisthesis (in which a spinal bone has slid forward out of position) or other back alignment problems. When a large section of bone has been removed due to an infection not relieved by antibiotics, a fusion can be done to increase back stability.

Fusions are unlikely to be done for a younger person in good health, or for an older person whose spine is characterized by rigidity. It is not useful for osteoporosis because the spinal bones are not solid enough to hold a graft.

Some back flexibility is lost by fusion, especially if two joints are fused instead of one. And when mobility is restricted in one area of the back, stresses can increase in other portions of the back. Fusion may result in different forces being exerted on the posterior facet joints as the spine's mechanics are changed.

BACK SURGERY RISKS

However unlikely they are to occur, risks should be explained to patients before surgery. Many knowledgeable people live with back pain due to structural defects rather than risk making the problem worse.

There are anesthesia risks, although these are extremely rare. A total of 1 to 2 percent of patients will develop a wound infection. The patient may be exposed to other hospital infections as well. Possible nerve damage or blood vessel damage could occur during surgery, along with pneumonia. Rarely, blood clots may travel to the lung during or after surgery.

The period of immobility following surgery, however brief, increases the possibility of blood clots, weakens muscles, and contributes to demineralization of bone. For at least a day or two before, during, and after surgery, the patient's nutritional needs are not met adequately.

PAIN MANAGEMENT

When pain can be managed in no other way, neurosurgeons can do surgery to interrupt nerve pathways to the brain. This may or may not resolve the problem. The understanding of pain remains incomplete. More likely at this time is the possible use of the TENS unit.

The use of a TENS unit, the acronym for transcutaneous electric nerve stimulation, involves the application of a continuous weak electrical current by way of electrodes placed on the skin. It may work by stimulating large nerve fibers, thus inhibiting transmission of pain signals or possibly, it is theorized, by increasing production of the body's own natural opiates. Those who have a pacemaker or heart disease do not wear a TENS unit.

Try acupuncture first.

CHAPTER TWELVE
KEEPING WHAT YOU'VE GOT

□

Having explored the pathways to total back fitness, you may wonder how all this will fit into your daily life. My approach has been to give guidelines, not a regimen. The focus of this book has been to give information with wide enough scope and perspective to assist you in making informed choices.

The underlying theme of this book has been that you "use it or lose it." Do a painting and it is done. On the other hand, your body is in a constant state of change, affected greatly by what you do or do not do. Back exercise brochures and classes and your doctors let you know, however hesitantly, that there is no end to these back exercises. The message is clear: Do them for the rest of your life.

This kind of commitment can sound a bit overwhelming if not impossible. Car maintenance, paying insurance bills, and tooth brushing and flossing can be managed; ignoring any of these results in known consequences. But a long-lasting commitment to exercise and body mechanics appears for many to be outside the realm of possibility. You do many helpful exercises and body positions automatically.

Because many—if not most—people stop doing back exercises when they recover and the pain goes away, maintenance strategies must be developed.

When or if back pain recurs, many just wait for the pain to recede while promising themselves that they will then resume those three or four back exercises on the sheet given them by their physicians. Yet, as the years pass, exercise becomes more, not less, important for bones, muscles, and joints. Suggestions in this chapter are designed to point you in this direction.

How can you avoid this dilemma and those unproductive guilt feelings? As with other health behavior changes, such as managing stress or changing eating habits, there are strategies that can help.

WHAT DO I HAVE TO DO?

First of all, some of the exercises in this book you will never adopt as your own. Any exercise or any sport doesn't do exactly for your body what any other exercise or sport can do. Whatever the substitutions, they are yours to make.

What you *have* to do depends on your goal.

"If I swim for twenty minutes twice a week my back doesn't hurt, but if I quit, then I get backaches again."

Another person says, "I used to get a lot of back pain, but now that I've started walking a mile each day my back feels fine."

This can sound almost like taking a magical potion, but what these two people are saying may be quite true.

An overwhelming commitment may not be required to avoid feeling back pain. What *is* required is a general pattern of consistency, several exercises several times a week, and a more or less constant background awareness of your body's comfort level and the stresses you may inadvertently be placing on it.

Whether what the above two people are saying will work depends on the particular situation of the individual's back and on *what else* is done all day or all week for back protection. Some people have adopted a lifestyle that tends to protect their backs.

The goal may be avoidance of pain, or it may be optimal back fitness. It may be somewhere in the middle of the spectrum. Your goals may change. After gaining control over backache and having the knowledge to proceed further, the temptation may be to give more exercise a try. Whatever your goal, it is easier to meet the goal you set than one imposed by others.

THE PROOF OF THE PUDDING

Does standing in a supermarket line for more than a few minutes leave you draped over the grocery cart and resting your elbows on the wire edges, even if the hour is not late? This experience may remind you of the discussion at the beginning of Level Three.

Does correct postural alignment require an inordinate amount of effort and attention? Do you get tired just trying to keep your rib cage up and your pelvis tilted? One of the rewards of a strong back (and most people still do not know that a strong back is both desirable and possible) is that correct postural alignment becomes easy and automatic. Improved appearance is a by-product of correct posture, a fact that is far from new. Doing a few curl-ups now and then is just not enough.

With a fit back there is less fear of injury, whether

jogging or attending an aerobics class. In diverse life-styles that might include involvement in contact sports, other active sports, prolonged sitting, or vehicular travel, a strong, flexible back and body are especially important. There are benefits to doing more than simply keeping your back discomfort below the pain threshold.

TO MAINTAIN, OR NOT TO MAINTAIN

"What are you doing for your back?"

"Nothing at the moment."

In the discussion of Level Three conditioning the point was made that you are, in fact, never doing "nothing." For better or for worse, you are maintaining your back. You may not see yourself clearly taking charge of your back and your body, but while moving through the day, minute by minute and hour by hour, what you do is low-risk or high-risk, helpful or not, including the car you ride in and the chair you sit in. What is involved is more a matter of self-care than one of time.

Doing even one thing for yourself can help. Get a better chair at home, such as a semireclining lounger with lumbar support to take the compression-loading forces off your spine.

Rocking chairs in the office are probably out of the question, but you might find a chair with a contoured seat that tilts backward to vary the angle of incline. At least find an office chair with armrests. If this is impossible, lean your elbows on your desk, keeping your back *straight*. Bring in a footstool to raise at least one knee above the level of your hips, or place one foot on the edge of an opened desk drawer, or on a wastebasket placed on its side.

Even if you have never in your life had a twinge of

back pain, buy a covered foam wedge for your chair and carseat that supports your back all the way to chest level (the thick part of the wedge is against your tail-bone and lower spine). Once in a while do a slow back arch followed by a pelvic tilt to give your spine some range of motion instead of keeping it "planted" in one position.

Comparing benefits and risks to your back at home and at work is hard. At home your general level of physical activity is often higher; of course, this depends on your occupation and how you spend your time at home. At home you can rest your back in the horizontal position at times. Both the rest and the activity are beneficial. What is lacking are muscle strengthening activities, including both the back muscles and the abdominals.

Hasty, inappropriate bending and lifting actions are possible risk behaviors at home. Vacuum cleaning is often hard on backs, with upright models usually producing less back strain. Bending over sinks, making beds, and all lifting activities require the ongoing use of information in this book.

Bending over your car engine without putting one foot on the bumper can strain your back; so can raking a yard or hoeing a garden. When sitting on a backless picnic table bench, keep your back straight, not hunched into a forward-bending position. At times rest your elbows on the edge of the table.

In the workplace the common risks are immobility or limited mobility with the back maintained fairly constantly in one position. Back and abdominal muscle tone can decline. Frequently there is associated muscle tension of back, shoulders, and neck. Research in Sweden on compression loading of the spine in various body positions showed that sitting is high on the list, almost the highest, in terms of disc pressure. Your challenge is monitoring feelings of back stiffness. Instead of tolerating them, develop strategies for response.

Change body position, however slightly. Walk at intervals, if only briefly. While you sit, stretch your back occasionally by bringing your shoulders toward your bent knees. Bring one knee at a time up toward your shoulders for a hamstring stretch.

Neck and shoulder tension can increase with the use of overhead fluorescent light. Use of a shaded desk lamp at or below eye level is often less stressful, and you may be less likely to hunch your shoulders over your work. Noise reduction is known to decrease overall body muscle tension and blood pressure as well. The field of ergonomics, concerned especially with workplace environmental health, has much to offer for increased comfort levels.

Vacations often present a special challenge because life-styles on vacations are often very different from life at home. If no efforts at all are made and the back is ignored, a vulnerable back can be placed at risk, but there always are steps you can take.

Travel often involves prolonged sitting, combined with the vibrational forces of vehicular travel, which are known, through occupational health research, to increase the stress on the structures of the back and to contribute to back pain. Another possible risk is that body weight may also increase. And, although you can skip a few days, remember that muscle tone (strength) begins to decline within a few days of inactivity.

But during vacations, maintenance of your back program can continue—the awareness of body comfort, attention to finding opportunities to walk, to stretch out body muscles, the continuance of back and abdominal exercises, and other self-selected exercises. Use hotel swimming pools and other exercise opportunities now available in many hotels.

Maintaining both a pain-free and a fit back involves selecting an ongoing exercise program and incorporating it, in a manner you choose, into your daily life. Succeeding sections of this chapter will give you additional guideposts for "keeping what you've got."

TRYING TOO HARD

Suppose we view an actor in a stage scene. Our actor, trying to do the most possible for his or her back, starts the day by leaping out of bed at the first sound of the alarm, whips through twenty-five bent-knee sit-ups, does a rapid series of twenty pelvic rocks, and throws in a few jumping exercises "to get the blood flowing." Our actor then drags out the trash and heads out for a brief run before embarking on a stop-and-start bus ride.

Despite our actor being active and doing exercises, this regime is hard on the back. The bouncing or jumping, especially in the morning with no warm-up, can be a real problem even for an apparently healthy back. Low-impact aerobics are replacing high-impact aerobics classes, and the same rationale applies to exercises done at home.

DOING IT RIGHT

Suppose, instead, that our stage actor wakes in more gentle fashion, does some slow, deep breathing and stretches before arising, and gets out of bed by first rolling to the side. This protects the back and avoids rising by doing a straight-knee sit-up, which may harm the back.

After arising, our actor does a few more favorite stretches in the standing position. The first conscious effort at muscular contraction is that of pulling in the abdomen before walking.

Our actor later does one or more repetitions of a few favorite exercises from Levels One, Two, and Three. Whether done on the bed or on the living room carpet, they are performed slowly, with attentive awareness of their effect on the body, and accompanied by deep, relaxing breathing.

Perhaps our actor will walk a few blocks or more before getting on the bus, or will get off the bus a few blocks before the destination.

TIME OUT FOR A BREATHING BREAK

Beverage breaks are accepted at home, school, work, and at meetings and conferences. They have become culturally legitimized and even legalized. The break can be used to help your back.

If you have been sitting, stand. Change the angle of your chair. Put your feet up (without resting your weight on the middle of your back). Stretch and take a few deep breaths. Do Benson's relaxation response (see Bibliography) and practice a couple of minutes of the relaxation techniques described earlier in this book. Your back muscles will relax, too.

Take the opportunity to talk or visit, or relax by yourself to clear your mind with serenity and seclusion.

TRY IT—YOU'LL LIKE IT

Levels One, Two, and Three exercises offer you an awesome inventory of exercise possibilities available in no other single source.

Try each, even if just once. Develop your skills in discovering what appears best for your back and your body. Only by finding out how each one feels can you know which ones may work best for you. Check out the effects on posture, and on muscles being stretched or shortened. Your continued commitment depends greatly on whether you do the ones that seem to enhance your feelings of well-being.

TAKE IT FROM HERE

To maintain a fit back, the following sequence is suggested. Substitute as you wish, based on what you have learned about what your back requires. Do the exercises from two to five times per week on a carpet or a mat, or on a bed if you prefer and if the mattress is firm. Perform one, two, several, or more repetitions of each, depending on your life-style, your athletic proficiency, and your comfort level. As stressed throughout this book, the benefits are maximized by slow, controlled repetitions, even if the exercise is done just once. Start with exercises based on the principles of the Williams flexion exercises.

1. Lying supine with knees raised, press the middle of your back against the carpet. Do the same with your knees apart.

2. Draw one knee at a time up toward your chest. Draw up both knees at once. Straighten your knees so that your legs are perpendicular to your body. Bring them apart, again together and down.

3. While still supine, tighten in your abdomen, tighten your buttocks, and raise your shoulders off the carpet or mat. Do the same, raising your feet and shoulders off the mat, with tight abdomen in the curl-up.

4. Do a total body stretch, still lying supine, with your pelvis maintained in a pelvic tilt.

To increase back fitness, do the following in light of increased attention to body stretches and warm-ups. Pick several from those described in preceding pages in addition to the preceding four. Presented here are three of them.

5. Stretch your calf muscles by standing with your feet flat on the floor and bending your knees until you feel the stretch.

6. Do a few shoulder circles and neck stretches.

7. While standing, do several lateral side bends.

Do several back exercises based on McKenzie principles as described in Level Three exercises in Chapter Eight.

8. Lie prone for a couple of minutes. Raise your straightened legs off the floor a few inches. Raise your shoulders off the floor. Then try both, lifting your legs and shoulders off the floor. Spread your legs into a "V" and release.

9. While supine, do the "three point" exercise in Level Three. Your weight is on your shoulders and heels.

10. Swim, using the crawlstroke.

Finally, for total back fitness pick an aerobic activity, whether walking, bicycling, swimming, or whatever you like. Do it for fifteen to twenty minutes at least two or three times per week, but not daily.

GOING THE EXTRA MILE

Described in these pages has been an extensive range of selected back care exercises, with the goal of total back fitness combined with discussion of the continuing unknowns, the controversies, and the medicine.

How much of the expected "normal" degenerative changes in the back can be delayed by the use of extensive back protection measures is unknown. Can protective measures combined with postural improvements and muscle strengthening including those of the back, possibly have a preventive effect on the aforedescribed degenerative changes in spinal bones and discs?

To date most efforts have, for obvious practical reasons, been limited to alleviating the immediate clinical problem of back pain. This has been challenge enough. Many—both back sufferers and exercise enthusiasts—have expressed the desire for more.

GLOSSARY

ABDUCTOR the muscle on the outside of the hipbone

ADDUCTOR the muscle of the inner thigh

CERVICAL SPINE the portion of the spinal column in the neck region

COCCYX the lowermost portion of the spinal column

DELTOID the muscle on top of the shoulders

DISC fibrous tissue with an inner core of gelatinlike material approximately ¼ to ¾ inches thick located between the spinal vertebrae and serving a shock-absorbing function

DISKECTOMY the surgical excision of the disc

ERECTOR SPINAE the longitudinal back muscles that straighten the back and are a frequent source of back pain

FACET the small flat surfaces on the spinal bones that permit the spinal bones to glide over each other when the back is in motion

GLUTEUS muscle of the buttocks

HAMSTRING the muscle in back of the thigh

LIGAMENT a strong, elastic band that holds a joint together, and that in the spine keeps vertebrae in place by binding discs and vertebral joints

LUMBAR VERTEBRAE the five weight-bearing vertebrae located between the thoracic vertebrae of the chest and the sacrum

OSTEOPHYTES extra bony growths on the vertebrae

OSTEOPOROSIS the condition of demineralization of the bones

PELVIC TILT the body position in which the abdominal muscles are contracted and the buttocks tucked down and under the spine

QUADRICEPS the muscle in the front of the thigh

SACRUM the lower portion of the spine below the lumbar region

SCIATIC NERVE the largest nerve in the body, located in the hip region and extending down the back of each thigh to the knee

SCOLIOSIS the sideways curvature of the spine

SPINAL COLUMN the column of individual bones (the vertebrae) that surround and protect the spinal cord and support the back

SPINAL CORD a network of nerve fibers that relay messages and sensations to and from the brain, running from the base of the skull through the spinal canal, the open portion of each vertebra.

SPINAL FUSION a surgical procedure using bone grafts to connect two or more vertebrae

TENDON the connective fibers attaching the muscles to bones

THORACIC the twelve vertebrae of the spine in the mid- and upper back where the ribs attach to the spine

TRACTION the use of weights to increase the separation between the vertebrae

TRANSITIONAL JOINT the abnormal joining of one lumbar vertebra to the adjoining vertebra on one side of the vertebral column

TRAPEZIUS   muscle of the upper back

VERTEBRA   one of the bones that in combination form the spine or backbone, permitting the erect stance, flexibility, and mobility

BACK ORGANIZATIONS

American Academy of Physical Medicine and Rehabilitation
30 North Michigan Avenue
Chicago, Illinois 60602
312-236-9512

American Medical Association
535 Dearborn Street
Chicago, Illinois 60611
312-645-5000

American Osteopathic Association
212 E. Ohio Street
Chicago, Illinois 60611
312-280-5800

American Physical Therapy Association
1111 N. Fairfax Street
Alexandria, Virginia 22314
703-684-2782

American Podiatry Association
20 Chevy Chase Circle, N.W.
Washington, D.C. 20015
202-537-4900

Arthritis Foundation
1314 Spring Street
Atlanta, Georgia 30309
404-872-7100

Clearinghouse for Occupational Safety and Health Information
4676 Columbia Parkway
Cincinnati, Ohio 45226
513-684-8326

U.S. Food and Drug Administration
Consumer Inquiry
5600 Fishers Lane
Rockville, Maryland 20852
301-443-3170

BIBLIOGRAPHY

TEXTBOOKS

Gray's Anatomy, 35th ed., by Warwick, Roger, M.D. and Williams, Peter, Dr. S. Edinburgh: Longman Group, Ltd., 1973.

Hadler, N. M. *Medical Management of the Regional Musculoskeletal Disease: Backache, Neck Pain, Disorders of the Upper and Lower Extremities.* Orlando, Fla.: Grune & Stratton, 1984.

Turek, Samuel. *Orthopedics,* 4th ed., vol. 2. Philadelphia: J. B. Lippincott, 1984.

Van De Graff, Kent, and Fox, Stuart Ira. *Concepts of Human Anatomy and Physiology.* Dubuque, Ia.: Wm. C. Brown, 1986.

OTHER BOOKS

Benson, Herbert, M.D. *The Relaxation Response.* New York: William Morrow & Company, 1975.

Berland, Theodore, and Addison, Robert, M.D. *Living with Your Bad Back.* New York: St. Martin's Press, 1972.

Chew, Robin Moquette; Brown-Machen, Marcia; Klatzky, Jennifer; Moquette, Elaine. *Fitness and Health Handbook.* Berkeley: University of California Press, 1985.

Fine, Judylaine. *Conquering Back Pain.* New York: Prentice Hall Press, 1987.

Friedmann, Laurence, M.D. *Freedom from Backaches.* New York: Simon & Schuster, 1973.

Hall, Hamilton, M.D. *The Back Doctor.* New York: McGraw-Hill, 1980.

Hatfield, Frederick C., Ph.D. *Bodybuilding: A Scientific Approach.* Chicago: Contemporary Books, 1984.

Keim, Hugo, M.D. *How to Care for Your Back.* Englewood Cliffs, N.J.: Prentice-Hall, 1981.

Kurland, Howard, M.D. *Back Pains: Quick Relief Without Drugs.* New York: Simon & Schuster, 1983.

Lettvin, Maggie. *Maggie's Back Book: Healing the Hurt in Your Lower Back.* Boston: Houghton Mifflin, 1976.

Linde, Shirley. *How to Beat a Bad Back.* New York: Rawson, Wade, 1980.

McKenzie, R. *The Lumbar Spine,* ed. 1. Upper Hutt, N.Z.: Wright and Carmen, Ltd., 1980.

Mellaby, Alexander. *The Y.M.C.A. Back Program. The Y's Way to a Healthy Back.* Piscataway, N.J.: New Century Publishers.

Noble, Elizabeth. *Essential Exercises for the Childbearing Year.* Boston: Houghton Mifflin, 1976.

———. *Marie Osmond's Exercises for Mothers-to-Be.* New York: New American Library, 1985.

———. *Marie Osmond's Exercises for Mothers and Babies.* New York: New American Library, 1985.

Powell, Don, Ph.D., and Singer, Carole, M. Ed. *Back at Work.* 1986. One of a series of health books by American Institute of Preventive Medicine, 19111 W. 10 Mile Road, Suite 101, Southfield, Mich. 48075.

Sarno, John, M.D. *Mind over Back Pain.* New York: William Morrow & Company, 1984.

Shuman, David, D.O. *Your Aching Back.* New York: George Staab, Gramercy Publishing, 1980.

Stoddard, Alan, M.D., D.O. *The Back: Relief from Pain.* New York: Arco Publishing, 1979.

Talman, William, M.D. *The No More Back Trouble Book.* Briarcliff Manor, N.Y.: Stein and Day, 1980.

Tarlov, Edward, D.O. and D'Costa, David. *Back Attack.* Boston: Little, Brown & Company, 1985.

Vickery, Donald, M.D. *Surviving the Hospital Experience.* Reston, Va.: The Center for Corporate Health Promotion, 1986.

White, Augustus A. III, M.D. *Your Aching Back.* New York: Boston Books, 1983.

Williams, P. *Low Back and Neck Pain: Causes and Conservative Treatment,* ed. 3. Springfield, Ill.: Charles C. Thomas, 1974.

JOURNAL ARTICLES

Aberg, J. "Evaluation of an Advanced Back Pain Rehabilitation Program." *Spine* 9, no. 3 (April 1984): 317–18.

Andersson, G. B. "Epidemiologic Aspects on Low Back Pain in Industry." *Spine* 6 (1981): 530–60.

Ballantyne, B.; Reser, M.; Lorenz, G.; and Schmidt, G. J. "The Effects of Inversion Traction on Spinal Column Configuration, Heart Rate, Blood Pressure, and Perceived Discomfort." *J. Orthopaedic and Sports Physical Therapy* 7, no. 15 (March 1986): 254–60.

Bennett, W. I., M.D. "Low Back Pain: What About Chiropractors?" *Harvard Medical School Health Letter* 13, no. 3 (January 1988).

Cappozzo, A. "Compressive Loads in the Lumbar Vertebral

Column During Normal Level Walking." *J. Orthopaedic Research* 1, no. 3 (1984): 292–300.

Castellvi, A., M.D.; Goldstein, L., M.D.; Chan, D., M.D. "Transitional Vertebrae and Their Relationship with Lumbar Extradural Defects." *Spine* 9, no. 5 (July–August 1984): 493–95.

Damkst, D. "The Relationship Between Work History, Work Environment, and Low Back Pain in Men." *Spine* 9 no. 4 (1984): 395–99.

Deyo, R. "Chymopapain for Herniated Intervertebral Discs." *Spine* 9, no. 5 (July–August 1984): 474–78.

Deyo, R.; Diehl, A.; and Rosenthal, M. "How Many Days of Bed Rest for Acute Low Back Pain? A Randomized Clinical Trial." *New England Journal of Medicine* 315, no. 17 (October 23, 1986): 1064–1107.

Fahmi, W. "Conservative Treatment of Lumbar Disc Degeneration: Our Primary Responsibility." *Orthop. Clin. North Am.* (1975): 93–103.

Gotfried, Y.; Bradford, D.; and Oegema, T. "Facet Joint Changes After Chemonucleolysis-Induced Disc Space Narrowing." *Spine* 11, no. 9 (1986): 944–49.

Gracovetsky, S., and Farfan, H. "The Optimum Spine." *Spine* 11, no. 6 (1986): 543–71.

Hadler, N., M.D. "Regional Back Pain." *New England Journal of Medicine* 315, no. 17 (October 23, 1986): 1090–92.

Hansson, T.; Bigos, S.; Wortley, M.; and Spengler, D. "The Load on the Lumbar Spine During Isometric Strength Testing. *Spine* 9, no. 7 (October 1984): 720–33.

Hayne, C. "Back Schools and Total Back Programmes: A Review." *Physiotherapy* 70, no. 1 (January 1984).

Hemborg, B.; Moritz, U.; Hemborg, H.; Holmstrom, E.; and Lowing, H. "Intra-abdominal Pressure and Trunk Muscle Activity During Lifting: Effect of Abdominal Muscle Training in Chronic Low Back Pain." *Scand. J. Rehab. Med.* 17, no. 1 (1985): 15–24.

Jayson, M.; Sims-Williams, H., Young, S.; Baddeley, H.; and

Collins, E. "Mobilization and Manipulation for Low-Back Pain." *Spine* 6 (1981): 490–95.

Jensen, R. "Disabling Back Injuries Among Nursing Personnel: Research Needs and Justification." *Res. Nurs. Health* 10, no. 1 (February 1987): 29–38.

Johnson, G. T., M.D. "Back Strain and Disc Problems." *Harvard Medical School Health Letter* 4: no. 5 (March 1979).

Kuo, P., and Loh, Z. "Treatment of Lumbar Intervertebral Disc Protrusion by Manipulation." *Clinical Orthopaedics and Related Research* 215 (February 1987): 47.

Lavsky-Shulan, M.; Wallace, R.; Kohout, F.; Lemke, J.; and Morris, M. "Prevalence and Functional Correlates of Low Back Pain in the Elderly." *J. Am. Ger. Assoc.* 33, no. 1 (January 1985): 23–28.

Lee, C., and Langran, N. "Lumbosacral Spinal Fusion." *Spine* 9, no. 6 (1984): 574–81.

McKenzie, R. "Prophylaxis in Recurrent Low Back Pain." *New Zealand Medical Journal* 89 (1979): 22–23.

Macnab, I. "Disc Degeneration and Low Back Pain." *Clinical Orthopaedics and Related Research* 208 (July 1986).

Maroon, J. C., M.D.; Orik, G., M.D.; and Day, A., M.D. "Percutaneous Automated Diskectomy in Athletes." *Physicians and Sportmedicine* 16, no. 8 (August 1988): 61.

Mather, D. "How to Move Patients the Easy Way—and Save Your Back." *Nursing* 17, no. 3 (March 1987): 55–57.

Mellin, G. "Treatment of Patients with Chronic Low Back Pain." *Scand. J. Rehab. Med.* 6, no. 2 (1984): 77–84.

Micheli, L. "Back Injuries in Dancers." *Clinical Sports Medicine* 22, no. 3 (November 1983): 473–84.

Miller, D. "Comparison of Electromyographic Activity in the Lumbar Paraspinal Muscles of Subjects with and without Low Back Pain." *Phys. Ther.* 65, no. 9 (September 1985): 1347–54.

Molumphy, M. "Incidence of Work-Related Low Back Pain in Physical Therapists." *Phys. Ther.* 65, no. 4 (April 1985): 482–86.

Nachemson, A. "The Lumbar Spine: An Orthopaedic Challenge." *Spine* 1 (1976): 59–71.

Ponte, D.; Jensen, G.; and Kent, B. "A Preliminary Report on the Use of the McKenzie Protocol Versus Williams Protocol in the Treatment of Low Back Pain." *J. Orthopaedic and Sports Physical Therapy* 6, no. 2 (September–October 1984): 130–39.

Prolo, D.; Oklund, S.; and Butcher, M. "Toward Uniformity in Evaluation Results of Lumbar Spine Operations: A Paradigm Applied to Posterior Lumbar Interbody Fusions." *Spine* 11, no. 6 (1986): 601–6.

Rosenthal, D. "CT in Diagnosis of Low Back Pain." *Applied Radiology* 14, no. 1 (January–February 1985): 163–68.

Schultz, A. B.; Warwick, D. N.; Berkson, M. H.; and Nachemson, A. L. "Mechanical Properties of the Human Lumbar Spine Motion Segments—Part I: Responses in Flexion, Extension, Lateral Bending, and Torsion." *J. Biomech. Eng.* 101 (1979): 46–52.

Sinaki, M.; McPhee, M.; Hodgson, S.; Merrit, J.; Offord, K. "Relationship Between Bone Mineral Density of the Spine and Strength of Back Extensors in Healthy Post-menopausal Women," *Mayo Clinic Proceedings* 61 (1986): 116–122.

Silberner, J., Budansky, S., Carey, J. and Wellborn, S. "Taking the Pain out of Pain." *U.S. News & World Report* (June 29, 1987): 50–56.

Sorensen, F., and Thomsen, C. "Medical, Social, and Occupational History as Risk Indicators for Low-Back Trouble in a General Population." *Spine* 11, no. 7 (1986): 721–23.

Sponseller, P.; Cohen, M.; Nachemson, A.; Hall, J.; and Wohl, E. "Results of Surgical Treatment of Adults with Idiopathic Scoliosis." *J. Bone and Joint Surgery* 69-A, no. 5 (June 1987): 667–74.

Thorstensson, A.; Carlson, H.; Zomleter, M. R.; and Nilsson, J. "Lumbar Back Muscle Activity in Relation to Trunk Movements During Locomotion in Man." *Acta Physiol. Scand.* 116 (1982): 13–20.

Troup, J. "Causes, Prediction, and Prevention of Back Pain at Work." *Scand. J. Work Envir. Health* 10, no. 6 (December 1984): 419–28.

Vijany, G.; Nishiyama, K.; Weinstein, J.; and Liu, Y. "Mechanical Properties of Lumbar Spinal Motion Segments as Affected by Partial Disc Removal." *Spine* 11, no. 10 (1986): 1008–12.

Waddell, G. "A Concept of Illness Tested As an Improved Basis for Surgical Decision in Low-Back Disorders." *Spine* 11, no. 7 (September 1986): 712–19.

Walker, J. "Age-Related Differences in the Human Sacroiliac Joint: A Histological Study; Implications for Therapy." *J. Orthopaedic and Sports Physical Therapy* 7, no. 6 (May 1986): 325.

Walloe, A., and Sunden, G. "Operations for Herniated Lumbar Discs: A Follow-Up Study 2–5 Years After Surgery." *Spine* 11, no. 6 (1986): 636–37.

Williams, P. "Examination and Conservative Treatment for Disk Lesions of the Lower Spine." *Clin. Orthop.* 5 (1955): 28–40.

INDEX

abdominal muscles, 48, 73,
   113, 138
   exercises for, 138–139
   separation of, checking for,
   73, 163
abductor muscle, 211
acupressure, 191
acupuncture, 191
adductor muscle, 211
aerobic exercise, 66–67, 145,
   147, 157, 164, 206
aging, 187
   bone loss and, 40, 45, 55,
   112
   disc problems and, 40–41
airplanes, sitting in, 102–103
alignment, spinal, 42–45, 48
   pelvic tilt and, 79–80
all fours with leg and arm
   extension, 134–135, 160
"amateur ice skater" stance,
   79–80, 107
American College of Sports
   Medicine, 145
American Heart Association, 66
American Institute for
   Preventive Medicine, 9
American Physical Therapy
   Association, 37
anesthesia, postpartum exercise
   and, 162
ankle circles, 120, 158

ankles, sprained, 49
anorexia nervosa, 49
arching of back, 74, 106–110
   prone position and, 21–22
arm extension on all fours,
   134–135, 160
arms, 49, 140
   rotation of, 119–120
arthritis, 44, 45, 187–188
   osteo-, 185–186, 196
   rheumatoid, 186
aspirin, 190

back:
   arching of, 21–22, 74,
   106–110
   extension exercises for, 106,
   108–110, 164
   flexing of, 74
   lying flat on, 20–21
   muscle groups of, 148–150
   protection of, daily activities
   and, 92–104
   stretching of, 57–59
   structure of, 36–47
   upper, 148, 213
back fitness, maintenance of,
   200–210
   exercise routine for, 208–209
back pain:
   causes of, 32–51
   description of, 17–18

back pain (*cont.*)
  diagnosis of, 171, 177–185
  disc problems and, 35–41
  eating disorders and, 49
  exercise programs and, 15
  facet joint misalignment and,
    46–47, 185–186
  incidence of, 9–10
  "irritated focus" of, 34
  issues and questions
    regarding, 10–16
  medical attention for,
    167–168
  medical responsiveness to,
    11, 12, 14–15
  muscle condition and, 48–49
  nerves and, 41–42, 167, 168,
    173
  patient response to, 10–16,
    50
  position for relief of, 63–64
  prevention of, 33, 36
  repetitive tasks and, 30,
    50–51
  risk factors associated with,
    10, 29–31
  sex and, 141–142
  strain and, 33–35
  stress and, 50
  systemic illness and, 189
  in tribal societies, 186
  upper back problems and, 49
  urinary problems and, 167
  weight and, 23, 29, 40, 109
back pain treatment:
  acupuncture for, 191
  aspirin for, 190
  biofeedback for, 191
  braces for, 61, 193
  casts for, 193
  chymopapain for, 195–196
  cold applications for, 24–25
  conservative, 15–16, 18,
    189–194
  corsets for, 61, 193
  disc excision for, 196–197
  "hanging" therapies for, 47,
    192–193
  heat applications for, 25,
    57–58
  laminectomy for, 197
  massage for, 191
  rest for, 190
  sex as, 141–142
  spinal fusion for, 173,
    197–198, 212
  sports and, 10
  supports for, 61–62
  surgical procedures for,
    194–199
  traction for, 191, 212
  weight loss for, 190
  see also bed rest; exercise
back protection, 92–104
  bending and, 94–98, 204
  lifting and, 98–100, 204
  sitting and, 101–103,
    204–205
  standing and, 93–94
  traveling and, 104
back strain, 33–35
back stretch exercises, 120,
  123–124
  side-lying, 57–59
balance chairs, 102
baseball, 153
basketball, 152
bed:
  changing positions in, 55–56
  reading position in, 22
bed board, 19
bed exercises, 57–61
bed making, 96–97
bed rest, 11, 19–24
  balance between exercise
    and, 52–54, 65–66
  caloric intake during, 23–24
  elderly and, 55
  lying positions during, 20–22
  planning for, 22–24
  pros and cons of, 54–55
bending, 94–98, 158, 204
Benson, Herbert, 59
bicycling, 152, 157
biofeedback, 191
body stretch, supine, 118–119
bone loss, 40, 45, 47, 55, 112,
  181, 186, 189, 194
bone scans, 183
bones, fracture of, 189

bowling, 152–153
braces, 61, 193
breaststroke, 133
breathing techniques, 56,
    60–61, 75–76
bridging, 108–109, 131
buttocks, muscles of, 148, 211
buttock walk, 139–140

calcium loss, 55
calves:
    muscles of, 148
    stretches for, 88–90, 129
cardiovascular conditioning, 66,
    143–144, 145
cars:
    getting into, 98
    lower back support in, 30,
        102–103
casts, 193
CAT scan, *see* CT scan
cervical spine, 211
Cesarean birth, 161–162
chairs, 29, 30, 101–103,
    203–204
    rocking, 101, 203
chest, muscles of, 148
chest stretches, 122–123
child back carriers, 165
childbirth:
    Cesarean, 161–162
    classes for, 155–156
    exercises for, 82–83,
        125–126, 158–160
chiropractors, 175–176
chymopapain, 195–196
coccyx, 211
contraction of muscle, 106, 111
Cooper, Kenneth, 66
corsets, 61, 193
crawl swimming stroke, 90, 91,
    133, 159
cribs, infant, 97–98
CT scan, 183–184
curl-ups, 83, 163
    diagonal, 139

deltoid muscle, 148, 211
diagnostic procedures, 171,
    177–185

questions about, 179–180
range of motion test for,
    178
disc excision, 196–197
discograms, 181–182
discs, 33–34, 35–41, 211
    aging of, 40–41
    herniation of, 37, 38, 40, 41,
        178
    rupture of, 36, 37–38, 40,
        41, 178
    slipped, 37, 38
disc spaces, narrowing of, 40,
    41
diskectomy, 196–197
diving, 154
"dowager's hump," 45
drinking fountains, 97

eating disorders, back pain
    and, 49
elderly, bed rest and, 55
electromyography, 181
endorphins, 146
erector spinae muscles, 112,
    148, 149, 211
estrogen, 194
exercise:
    aerobic, 66–67, 145, 147,
        157, 164, 206
    after pregnancy, 160–165
    back extension versus flexion,
        108–110
    back strengthening,
        prerequisites for, 110–113
    back stretch, 57–59, 120,
        123–124
    balance between rest and,
        52–55, 65–66
    bed, 57–61
    benefits of, 65–67
    bone loss retardation and, 55,
        112
    breathing technique with, 56,
        60–61, 75–76
    during pregnancy, 82–83,
        108–109, 125–126,
        157–160, 164
    endorphin production and,
        146

exercise (*cont.*)
  flexion, 44, 106, 108–110,
    208
  high-intensity, 146
  lack of, back pain and, 10
  questions about, 66–69
  surgery vs., 12
  warm-ups and stretches
    before, 116–118
  warnings about, 77, 94
  weight-bearing, 55
exercise equipment, 143,
  144–145
  for aerobic conditioning,
    145
  use of, 146–150
exercises, bed, 57–61
exercises, Level One, 64–65
  back-lying pelvic tilt, legs
    extended, 74–75, 159, 163
  back pain relief position,
    64–65
  head raises, 72–73
  pelvic tilt all fours, 73–74,
    159, 163
  raised knee pelvic tilt, 71–72
  raised knee pelvic tilt with
    contracted buttocks, 72
  side-lying squat with
    tightened abdominals,
    70–71
  standing pelvic tilt, 76, 163
exercises, Level Two, 80–90
  bent-knee sit-ups, 80–81
  bent-knee sit-ups with knees
    apart, 81–82, 164
  calf stretch, 88–90
  curl-ups, 83, 163
  Kegel, 82–83, 158, 162
  knee-to-chest lower-back
    stretch, 80
  leg raises, 85–88
  pelvic floor, 82–83
  wall slides, 83–85, 159, 163
exercises, Level Three,
    strengthening, 130–141
  all fours with leg and arm
    extension, 134–135, 160
  buttock walk, 139–140

diagonal curl-ups, 139
diagonal sit-ups, 138–139
inner thigh tightening, 141
modified push-ups, 140, 160
prone head and shoulder
  raise, 135
prone leg raise, 135–136
prone lying, 130
sculling in water, 140–141
sex as, 141–142
standing back, 131–133
swimming, 133
"three point," 136–137
wagging your tail, 140
waist, legs, and hips, 141
walking, 130
exercises, Level Three,
    stretching, 118–129
  ankle circles, 120, 158
  back, 120, 123–124
  chest, 122–123
  inner thigh, 125
  inverted "V," 129
  neck, 121
  rotational, 124
  rotation of arms and legs,
    119
  shoulder circles, 121
  side-lying hip and back,
    119
  standing quad, 126–129
  standing side, 126
  standing squat, 125–126
  standing trunk rotation, 126
  supine body, 118–119
extend, extension, 45, 106

facet joints, 46–47, 185–186,
  211
family physicians, 176
fitness instructors, 145
flex, flexing, 106
flexion exercise, 106, 108–110,
  208
  definition of, 44, 106
fluorescent light, 205
fractures:
  of bones, 189
  of vertebrae, 45–46, 181

gastrocnemius muscle, 148
gluteal muscles, 148, 211
golf, 152
gyms, *see* health clubs

hamstring, definition of, 211
"hanging" therapies, 47,
    192–193
head and shoulder raise, prone,
    135
head raises, 72–73
health care providers:
    responsiveness of, 11, 12,
        14–15
    types of, 168, 172–177
health clubs, 143–150
    instructors at, 145
    selection of, 145–146
health insurance, 168–169,
    175, 176
health maintenance
    organizations (HMOs),
        168
heart attacks, exercise and, 66
heart rates, target, 145
heat, muscle relaxation and, 25,
    57–58
height, loss of, 40
herniated discs, 37, 38, 40, 41,
    178
hips:
    abduction of, 148, 211
    breaks in, 189
    side-lying stretch for, 119
    strengthening exercise for,
        141
HMOs (health maintenance
    organizations), 168
hormones:
    estrogen, 194
    relaxin, 40, 156–157
horseback riding, 152
hospitals:
    diagnostic procedures in,
        179–185
    emergency rooms of, 169
hot tubs, 157
hydroculator, 25
hyperextension, 44, 106

ice applications, 24–25
inner thigh, 211
    stretch for, 125
    tightening of, 141
insurance, health, 168–169,
    175, 176
internists, 173
"irritated focus" of back pain,
    34

Jacobsen, Edmund, 59
jogging, 151, 157
joints, 106, 212
    facet, 46–47, 185–186, 211
    sacroiliac, 36
    transitional, 212

Kegel exercise, 82–83, 158,
    162
knees, bending of, 21, 48–49,
    77, 95–96

laminectomy, 197
latissimus dorsi muscles, 148
legs:
    extension of, on all fours,
        134–135, 160
    raises, 77, 85–88, 135–136
    rotation of, 119–120
    strengthening exercise for,
        141
    stretches for, 129
    upper, muscles of, 149
Lettvin, Maggie, 58
lifting, 30, 58, 62, 98–100, 204
    rules for, 100
ligaments:
    definition of, 35, 211
    posterior longitudinal, 39–40
lower-back:
    stretch, knee-to-chest, 80
    swayback position of, 42
lumbar vertebrae, 212
lying positions, 20–22

McKenzie, Robin, 79, 108,
    109
magnetic resonance imaging
    (MRI), 184–185

massage, 191
mattress, 19
Mayo Clinic, 112
medical care, 11–13, 14–15,
    166–199
  diagnosis and, 177–185
  need for, 167–168
  sources of, 168–172
  specialists for, 168, 172–177
MRI (magnetic resonance
    imaging), 184–185
muscles, 47–49
  abdominal, 48, 73, 113,
    138–139, 163
  abductor, 211
  adductor, 211
  for back strength, 148–150
  of buttocks, 148, 211
  of calves, 148
  of chest, 148
  contraction of, 106, 111
  deltoid, 148, 211
  erector spinae, 112, 148,
    149, 211
  gastrocnemius, 148
  gluteal, 148, 211
  latissimus dorsi, 148
  of legs, 149
  quadriceps, 83–85, 126–129,
    159, 163, 212
  relaxation of, 25, 57–58,
    59–61
  repetitive use of, 30, 50–51
  shortening of, 21, 35
  of shoulders, 148, 211
  strengthening of, 21–22,
    146–148, 149–150
  stretching of, 106, 111,
    116–129
  tension and release of, 56,
    60–61
  thigh, 83–84, 125, 141, 211,
    212
  trapezius, 148, 213
  weakening of, 25
myelograms, 182–183

neck, 205
  positioning of, 103–104
  stretching exercises for, 121

nerves, 167
  sciatic, 41–42, 71, 168, 173,
    212
neurologists, 172
neuroradiologists, 174
neurosurgeons, 172
*New England Journal of
    Medicine,* 40
Noble, Elizabeth, 73
noise reduction, 205
numbness, 49, 168
nursing staffs, 177

orthopedists, 172
osteoarthritis, 185–186, 196
osteomyelitis, 188
osteopathy, 174
osteophytes, 181, 212
osteoporosis, 40, 45, 47, 55,
    112, 181, 186, 189, 194,
    212

pain, back, *see* back pain; back
    pain treatment
pain management, 197
pectoral muscles, 148
pelvic floor exercise, 82–83,
    158, 162
pelvic tilt, 70, 79–80
  definition of, 106, 212
  overly pronounced, 107, 108
pelvic tilt exercises:
  on all fours, 73–74, 159, 163
  back-lying, legs extended,
    74–75, 159, 163
  raised knee on back, 71–72
  raised knee on back with
    contracted buttocks, 72
  standing, 76, 163
physiatrist, 174–175
physical therapists, 176
physicians, family, 176
pillows, 20, 104
pregnancy, 73, 155–157
  disc rupture during, 40
  exercising after, 160–165
  exercising during, 82–83,
    108–109, 125–126,
    157–160, 164
X rays during, 12

prone leg raises, 135–136
prone position, 21–22
    definition of, 106
    as strengthening exercise,
        130
push-ups:
    modified, 140, 160
    straight-leg, 77

quadriceps, 212
    strengthening of, 83–85, 159,
        163
    stretch of, standing, 126–129

radiologist, 174
range of motion diagnostic test,
    178
reading in bed, 22
relaxation response, 30, 59–62
relaxin hormone, 40, 156–157
repetitive motions, back pain
    and, 30, 50–51
rheumatoid arthritis, 186
risk factors, back pain, 10,
    29–31
rocking chairs, 101, 203
rotational stretches, 124
rowing, rowing machines, 145,
    153–154
running, long-distance, 41
ruptured discs, 36, 37–38, 40,
    41, 178

sacralization, 45, 181
sacroiliac joint, 36
sacrum, 212
sailing, 153
sciatic nerve, 41–42, 71, 168,
    173, 212
scoliosis, 45, 173, 181, 187,
    212
sculling in water, 140–141
sex, 141–142
shoes, 29, 88, 93
    tying of, 98
shoulder circles, 121, 158
shoulders, 205
    and head raise, prone, 135
    muscles of, 148, 211
    strength, exercise for, 140

shoveling, 37
side, lying on, 21
side-lying back stretch, 57–59
side-lying hip and back stretch,
    119
side-lying squat, 70
side stretches, standing, 126
sitting, 29, 41, 76, 78,
    101–103, 115, 158,
    204–205
sit-ups:
    bent-knee, 80–81
    bent-knee with knees apart,
        81–82, 164
    diagonal, 138–139
    straight-leg, 77
skiing, 153
sleeping positions, 20–22
slipped disc, 37, 38
specialists, back, 168, 172–177
spinal cord, 41, 212
spinal fusion, 173, 197–198,
    212
spinal manipulation therapy,
    191
spinal X rays, 12–13, 175,
    180–181
spine, spinal column, 42–46,
    212
    alignment of, 42–45, 48,
        79–80
    cervical, 211
    conditions of, 45–46
    structure of, 42–45, 211,
        212
spondylitis, 187–188
spondylolisthesis, 188, 198
spondylolysis, 188
sports, 150–154, 157
    back pain and, 10
    injury from, 150
    see also specific sports
sprains, 33, 35, 49
standing, 29, 30, 53, 76, 78,
    93–94, 158
    locked knees and, 21
standing back exercise,
    131–133
standing leg raises, 86–88
standing squat stretch, 125–126

stenosis, 186–187
straight-leg raises, 77
strain, back, 33–35
stress:
    back pain and, 50
    management of, relaxation as,
        30, 59–62
stretch, back, 57–59
stretching, muscle, 116–118
    definition of, 106, 111
    exercises for, 118–129
    supine body stretch, 118–119
supine position, 20–21
    definition of, 106
surgery, 13, 166, 167, 168,
        170, 177
    exercise vs., 112
    pain management through,
        198–199
    pros and cons of, 194–199
    risks of, 198–199
    see also back pain treatment
swimming, 67, 68, 90–91, 157,
        159
    as strengthening exercise,
        133, 140

target heart rates, 145
Taylor, Andrew, 174
teeth, brushing of, 98
tendons, definition of, 35,
        212
tennis, 151
thigh muscles, 83–84, 211,
        212
    inner, stretch for, 125
    inner, tightening of, 141
thoracic vertebrae, 212
"three point" exercise,
        136–137
toe-touching exercise, warning
        about, 77, 94
traction, 192, 212
tranquilizers, 190–191
transitional joint, 212
trapezius muscle, 148, 213
travel, tips for, 104

tribal societies, back pain
        incidence in, 186
trunk rotation, standing, 126
tying of shoes, 98

ultrasound, 184
upper back, 148, 213
    muscles of, 148
    pain in, 49
upper body, exercise for,
        140–141
urinary problems, back pain
        and, 167

vacations, 205
vertebrae:
    fractures of, 45–46, 181
    lumbar, 212
    thoracic, 212

wagging your tail exercise, 140
waist, waistline:
    bending from, 94–95
    exercises for, 140, 141
walking, 67, 76, 78, 157, 160,
        162
    as strengthening exercise,
        130
wall slides, 83–85, 159, 163
warm-ups, 116–117
water beds, 19–20
weight, overweight:
    back exercises for, 109
    back problems and, 23, 29,
        40, 109
    loss of, as treatment, 168,
        190
weight-bearing exercise,
        calcium loss and, 55
weight lifting, 149–150
whirlpools, 157
White, Augustus A., III, 150
Williams, Paul, 79, 108, 109
writing implements, bed rest
        and, 26

X rays, 12–13, 175, 180–181

**Monroe County
Community College
Monroe, Michigan**

PRINTED IN U.S.A.

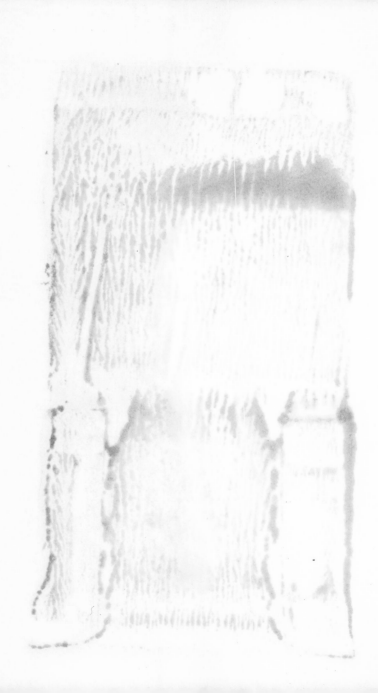